Springer Series on ADULTHOOD and AGING

Series Editor: Bernard D. Starr, Ph.D.

Advisory Board:
Paul D. Baltes, Ph.D., Jack Botwinick, Ph.D., Carl Eisdorfer, M.D., Ph.D.,
Donald E. Gelfand, Ph.D., Lissy Jarvik, M.D., Ph.D., Robert Kastenbaum, Ph.D.,
Neil G. McCluskey, Ph.D., K. Warner Schaie, Ph.D., Nathan W. Shock, Ph.D.,
and Asher Woldow, M.D.

Rosemary McCaslin, Ph.D., A.C.S.W., is Assistant Professor at the University of Texas at Austin, School of Social Work, and has been involved in the field of aging since 1972. She was formerly Director, Senior Information Service, Texas Research Institute of Mental Sciences in Houston, Texas. While in that position, Dr. McCaslin introduced elderly paraprofessional workers into the geriatric mental health team. This practice, considered unusual at its initiation, continues in the present as a strong component of the institute's program.

THE OLDER PERSON AS A MENTAL HEALTH WORKER

Rosemary McCaslin, Ph.D., A.C.S.W.
Editor

Springer Publishing Company
New York

Springer Publishing Company, Inc.
200 Park Avenue South
New York, New York 10003

83 84 85 86 87 / 10 9 8 7 6 5 4 3 2 1

Library of Congress Cataloging in Publication Data

Main entry under title:
The older person as a mental health worker.
  (The Springer series on adulthood and aging ; 12)
  Bibliography: p.
  Includes index.
   1. Aged in mental health—United States. 2. Aged—Mental health services—United
States. 3. Mental health services—United States. I. McCaslin, Rosemary. II. Series.
[DNLM: 1. Mental health services—In old age. 2. Voluntary workers. SP685N v.12 /
WM 30 044]
RC440.6.04 1983   362.2'0425   82-25632
ISBN 0-8261-4290-7

Printed in the United States of America

*This book is dedicated to the three older workers
who have taught me the most: my parents,
Miriam and James B. McCaslin, and Leonora Driver.*

Contents

Foreword

The chapters in this volume describe modest efforts in daily practice and may seem marginal when compared with the mainstream of scientific gerontology. We should, however, understand them as signs of an incipient and most needed epistemological and moral revolution. For these chapters tell us of older persons being called, and treated, as partners in the service of older people. These experiences may well not be the only ones along these lines or even not the first. But it is important that a book focus on such experiences.

The twentieth century, in launching gerontology, is the first period in history to view aging, old age, and older people as objects of scientific knowledge. Whether the abundant production in the field over the past four decades has resulted in a better understanding and management of human aging is at best doubtful, and the quality, theoretical status, scope, aim, object, and method of gerontology is still debatable. But there is no doubt that the new view has efficiently changed something in our society. A set of social institutions officially devoted to research and teaching on aging has been developing under the new label: institutes, centers, societies, conventions and colloquiums, academic programs and positions, chairs and professorships, fees, dues, stipends and grants, specialized journals and books. An aspect of this social change is that for the first time in history a few thousand individuals make a living in research and teaching on aging, or in investigating and teaching the aged.

Before the emergence of gerontology as a scientific study, people had not ignored aging. Everywhere and throughout history, old age and aging have been objects of experience, discussion, observation, specula-

tion, management, contempt or pity or fear or veneration, of stereotypes and fantasies, of endless discourses. It seems that in promoting
gerontology as a scientific undertaking its pioneers wanted to substitute
for all these former discourses, disregarded as prescientific, a sound,
verified, and reliable knowledge. The very ambition of building on new
grounds an entirely new knowledge may be regarded as the reverse of,
or the disguise of a refusal to validate, all that people had formerly
thought on the subject and the actual experience of aging as expressed
by the aged. With the development of what is called educational
gerontology, which encompasses both teaching on aging and teaching
the aged, we now have gerontologists, not yet retired, earning their
daily bread by teaching their elders what aging is. But the scientific
knowledge of aging is divorced from personal experience and from the
interpretation by which we give it a meaning.

In Plato's *Republic* Socrates tells us that we ought to enquire of
older people, as of travellers who have taken a journey that we too may
have to take, whether the way is smooth and easy or rugged and
difficult. Whether we know it or not, from childhood on we internalize
images of our elders as cues and patterns of the stages of our own future
development. These images are colored by emotions and feelings, so
that our plans and projects for our own futures are linked to fantasies
fears, and expectations. These images are also inevitably modified by
notions and criteria that we internalize from hearsay; they combine to
give us biased, abstract, misleading, and contradictory notions of the
ages of life. Our own experience of life, our experience of growth and
aging, will not necessarily correct these preconceptions and prejudices
because (1) they being loose and contradictory, we switch from one to
another according to circumstances and find in ambiguous reality
enough support to confirm our partial views, and (2) many of the traits
that characterize a given age of life result not from nature but from
social conventions and stereotypes, so that the prejudices create the
conditions of their own confirmation, act as self-fulfilling prophecies,
and are inevitably mistaken for natural phenomena and universal
laws.

The dialogue between Socrates and the old Cephalus, which is
developed in the Prologue of Plato's *Republic*, shows clearly that the
aged are considered and treated by Socrates as needed partners in a
shared, ongoing research, not as masters whose pronouncements
should be uncritically accepted as truth. To protect our own life we

cannot dispense with the experience of our elders, we must enquire from them. Our abstract notions will not do.

But their abstract notions will not do either. Their experience must be critically examined, and their own spontaneous formulation of it may well be inadequate. Actually, Socrates could not have asked "Is the way of old age smooth or rugged?" if he had not heard some old people praise, and others blame, old age; if he had not already formed the assumption that some people age well and some not; if he himself had not ambivalent notions, feelings, and expectations of old age. In enquiring of Cephalus, he asks what is the experience of Cephalus, which is different from that of other older people. The object of his question is, can we, by critical examination and comparative analysis of the varying patterns of human aging, assess the conditions that may help us to keep growing, or to find satisfactions or compensations when growing old, and sort them out from those that make aging rugged and difficult?

We shall never know what really is universal in human aging as long as we have not explored the full range of its variations in pace, effects, patterns, and styles, across cultures and throughout history. But what we must explore is the range not only of the variations that may have occurred and may have been observed and interpreted in the past. We must also explore the range of *potential* variations in human aging. These we can explore either by art and fiction, inasmuch as works of art offer to humanity models of feelings, attitudes, virtues, and behaviors that humans will by imitation embody and turn into historical reality, or by action, i.e., intervention, be it therapeutic, educational, social, technical, or political. Geriatrics and social policies for the aged have already contributed to change the living conditions, the social status, the cultural image of older people, old age, and aging. Far from solving the problems of the aged, they in some ways aggravate them. We must not think that scientists will build a scientific knowledge of aging and old age by observing "natural" processes of human aging without interfering in them, and that, on that basis, practitioners, physicians, nurses, social workers, educators, and policy makers will develop "applied gerontology." If today's knowledge of physiology may amend or arm medical intervention, we must not forget that it developed through, and grew out of, medical intervention. By collective and individual decisions and activities we keep on interfering with our own and others' aging. Experiential gerontology is already developing. How must we use such activities to amend our knowledge, to correct our misunderstandings, of human aging, knowing that not only will we *not* control all the variables, but that these activities must obey norms that are ethical, political, religious, economic, ideological, and not only "scientific"?

From this perspective active engagement of older workers in the service of older people must be hailed as an important and potentially fecund innovation in the management and service of the aged, in the interpretation of aging, and ultimately in our understanding of human aging. Through such patterns of intermingling the roles of expert and client, helper and helped, it becomes possible to draw on the knowledge that is uniquely held by the former "objects" of gerontological study. The expertise of both young and old becomes available and we are in a better position to discover how the path of aging may be made smoother for all people. In the process, we reaffirm the truth that it is people, whether gerontologists or lay persons, who must create their own solutions to the natural problems of life.

Michel Philibert
Director
Interdisciplinary Gerontology Center
University of Grenoble
Grenoble, France

Acknowledgments

The idea for this book began in a paper session at the Tenth International Congress of Gerontology in Jerusalem, in 1975, at which both McCaslin and Blumensohn presented papers and Philibert was present as a discussant. A lively and learned discussion followed the papers in which the benefits accruing to older persons through participation in the provision of human services was soundly endorsed. However, an appreciation of the other side of the coin seemed to be strangely lacking among most of those present, in spite of their considerable experience with the elderly. As the session ended, several of the participants realized that no consideration had been given to the strengths of older people that could (and should) be tapped by mental health enterprises. This book has been written in the hopes that future discussions will more readily consider both sides of the issue and that perhaps, there will be more older workers engaged in the discussions.

All of the contributors to this volume are indebted to a large number of persons who provided assistance, advice, and support. The traditional listing would probably constitute a chapter in and of itself. Most of us became involved in efforts to utilize older workers and volunteers before it was fashionable and have fought many long and difficult battles to convince funders and decision makers of the soundness of this idea. In the process, there can be no doubt that our most important source of ideas for new, productive program directions, our most important teachers as we refined our program designs, and our most valuable evidence in proving that these programs were worth support have been the individual older workers and volunteers with whom we have had the good fortune to collaborate. So in lieu of a list of acknowledgments, I shall take the liberty of expressing for all the contributors our deepest respect and admiration for the older persons who have had the courage to turn their backs on the stereotypes of old age and work with us on behalf of those persons of all ages who do need the assistance of capable and caring people.

Contributors

Ruth M. Bakke, R.N., M.S.N., is Interim Dean, College of Science and Technology, and Director, Nursing Program at Corpus Christi State University, Texas.

Leo Blumensohn is Project Director, The National Insurance Institute of Israel, Counseling Centers for Senior Citizens.

Elizabeth Bristowe, M.A., is Consultant on Gerontology, Ministry of Health, Province of British Columbia.

George A. Brown, A.C.S.W., is Director, West Philadelphia Corporation. He was formerly, Director of Base Service Unit and Counseling Centers, West Philadelphia Community Mental Health Consortium, Inc.

Herbert Diamond, M.D., is Medical Director, West Philadelphia Community Mental Health Consortium, Inc., and Associate Professor of Psychiatry, University of Pennsylvania School of Medicine.

Ernestine Estes, A.C.S.W., is Director, Specialized Programs, West Philadelphia Community Mental Health Consortium, Inc.

N. Claire Kowalski, M.S.W., is Assistant Professor of Human Development, Counseling and Family Studies, University of Rhode

Island. She was formerly Field Gerontologist, University of Rhode Island Program in Gerontology.

Judith Schapiro, Ed.D., is Professor/Chairperson, Department of Child Study and Special Education, Darden School of Education, Old Dominion University, Virginia.

Joan Walsh Trelease, R.N., M.A., is Director of Staff Development, Cranston General Hospital, Osteopathic, Cranston, Rhode Island.

Michael P. Tristan, M.D., M.P.H., is Assistant Professor, Departments of Community Medicine, Pediatrics, and Psychiatry, Baylor College of Medicine, Texas.

Nancy Wilson, M.A., is Long Term Care Channeling Project Site Director, Texas Research Institute of Mental Sciences, Gerontology Center. She was formerly Supervisor, Senior Information and Outreach Service, Texas Research Institute of Mental Sciences.

Part I
Introduction

1

Introduction

Rosemary McCaslin

... the right way to handle the old is to stop treating them as a problem when they are in fact a resource ...

(Comfort, 1977)

Western society has an unfortunate talent for creating "Catch 22s" in public policy—situations in which the response to a problem precludes its solution. A prime example of these no-win approaches can be seen in the underutilization of the skills and talents of older persons. Mental health problems are created for many older persons by policies of forced retirement while the mental health system is handicapped in its capacity to meet their needs because it lacks sufficient human resources for many roles that could be well filled by older workers. The situation feeds into what Comfort (1977) calls *sociogenic aging*—the role which our folklore, prejudices, and misconceptions about age impose on the old—and is obviously detrimental to persons of all ages.

In the United States today, only 12 percent of all persons aged 65 and over (2.5 million persons) are employed. Of those who are retired, 37 percent (4.4 million) feel they were forced to stop working and 31 percent of the elderly who are retired or unemployed (4 million) express a desire to work. Fifteen percent of the latter feel that lack of opportunities keeps them from working and 11 percent of all elderly feel they possess skills that they have no chance to use.

Whether employed or not, 4.5 million persons aged 65 and over (22 percent) contribute their skills and time in volunteer roles, most prominently in the areas of health and mental health (23 percent),

3

transportation (21 percent), civic affairs (17 percent), psychological and social support services (17 percent), distribution of in-kind assistance (16 percent), and family-, youth-, and child-oriented services (15 percent). An additional 10 percent of the elderly would like to be involved in volunteer services with 8 percent of these feeling that opportunities are not available to them (Harris, 1975).

These same older persons suffer from a disproportionate incidence of mental health problems. The President's Commission on mental Health (1978) estimates that up to 25 percent of persons aged 65 and over are mentally ill or emotionally disturbed as compared with 15 percent of the general population. Some of these disorders are associated with age-related arteriosclerotic and senile brain changes. It is also recognized, however, that a variety of somatic and environmental stresses—and especially depression—can masquerade as or exacerbate organic brain syndromes in the elderly (e.g., Gaitz, 1972; Kahn et al., 1975; Varner, 1976; Varner and Calvert, 1974). Older persons who are involuntarily retired may be prime candidates for depression as they face the loss of a significant activity which has long served to provide financial security, structure their time, define their status in the community, facilitate peer relations, and give a sense of meaning to their lives (Friedmann and Havighurst, 1954). Retirement itself, producing changes in numerous life areas affecting identity and self-esteem at the same time that it brings financial constraints on a person's ability to seek out alternatives for meeting such needs, is a major mental health problem in the lives of many older persons. The impact of such stresses is underscored by the fact that 25 percent of all suicides in the United States are committed by persons 65 and over.

At the same time that this pool of unused human resources exists, the mental health system is hard pressed to meet the service needs of the population. It is estimated that in the United States today there are 2 million schizophrenics, 1 million persons with organic psychoses, 10 million alcoholics, and 6 million mentally retarded persons. Twenty-five percent of the population is estimated to suffer from a variety of emotional disorders, 1 percent from depressive disorders, and 5–15 percent of children aged 3–15 from handicapping mental disorders. Yet in 1975 only 6.7 million persons, 3 percent of the American population, were seen in the specialized mental health sector and only 1.5 million persons were hospitalized in mental health facilities (President's Commission, 1978).

The recent report of the President's Commission on Mental Health concludes that the problem is not one of lack of mental health services.

Rather, the difficulties lie in the range, appropriateness, and acceptability of those which are available. While we have succeeded in moving mental patients from isolation in state hospitals back to a community-based environment, we have failed to provide the concomitant social and vocational services that are necessary if such persons are to function as part of the community. Such support services have not been traditionally supplied by the mental health system nor is it currently equipped to provide them. It has been assumed that these generic supports would be supplied by families and friends and the informal support networks of the community to which patients were returned. Yet little attention has been given to the strain that the reorganized mental health system would place on the resources of these community networks. The President's Commission now calls for efforts to bolster and integrate nonprofessional but essential daily life maintenance services within the mental health system.

Additionally, the President's Commission has pointed to the continued existence of underserved populations—ethnic and racial minorities, women, the aged. Here the problem is one of lack of cultural relevance of existing services. Efforts must continue to include the perspective of the potential client in planning, developing, and delivering services.

In a climate of fiscal conservatism and reluctance among taxpayers to bear the cost burden for public services, it is unclear how the personnel needs for these improvements in an already labor-intensive field such as mental health are to be financed. In 1976, the direct cost of mental health services in the United States was $17 billion, 12 percent of all health costs (President's Commission, 1978). The time has come, as Sarason and Lorentz (1979) have tried to impress on us, to reconsider the assumptions behind our resource allocation patterns and to think creatively about more efficient approaches. One avenue deserving further consideration is the use of indigenous paraprofessional workers. The social experiments of the 1960s provided a large body of literature which analyzes the benefits and difficulties of this approach (e.g., Austin, 1978; Barker and Briggs, 1968; Cohen, 1976; DHEW, 1974; Epstein, 1962; Gershon and Biller, 1977; Grosser, Henry, and Kelly, 1969; Heyman, 1966; Kent, Hirsch, and Barg, 1971; Richan, 1961, 1969, and 1972; Weed and Denham, 1961). It is widely concluded that (1) indigenous workers possess attributes and skills that are of value to the mental health field, (2) paraprofessionals can be trained to provide needed mental health services, and (3) the use of paraprofessionals can facilitate greater efficiency in the use of more expensive professional services. Additionally, paraprofessional careers have been seen as a mechanism for assisting persons with lower levels of education in escaping from cycles of chronic unemployment and underemployment, thus make a major indirect contribution to their own mental health.

Since the largest impetus for expanded use of paraprofessionals came from the War on Poverty, we have come to associate the term "indigenous worker" with the situation in which poor, unskilled persons are trained to assist their poor, unskilled neighbors. The concept is much broader, however, encompassing any attempt to match worker and client on major cultural characteristics in order to take advantage of the worker's "native" understanding of the cultural context of the client's difficulties. Certainly advanced age is an appropriate characteristic for such worker/client matching when the problem to be worked is related to physical, social, or psychological ramifications of growing older. Also, older persons may be utilized for their indigenous understanding in other areas such as race and class, and their vast experience, which may be in mental health or related fields, can be drawn upon.

A related service delivery concept that lends itself to the inclusion of older people and that is attracting increased attention as program funds become scarcer is the support and augmentation of natural support networks (Caplan and Killilea, 1976; Collins and Pancoast, 1977). Like the use of paraprofessionals, networking attempts to make use of the innate helping capacities of a broad range of people and to integrate the need to contribute to one's community with the need to receive assistance. Networking is less formal, less intrusive, and less costly than the creation of new job opportunities. It has been argued that it is more effective in maintaining achieved roles and status because it augments already established functions rather than requiring an untrained person to move into the alien professional world (Collins and Pancoast, 1977).

Older persons who do work and/or volunteer are often involved in the provision of health, mental health, and social services. Agencies and institutions that have tried utilizing older workers and volunteers have found many to possess a "people sense" acquired through life experience and a patience derived from having fewer demands made on one's time which lend themselves well to carrying out the labor-intensive basic caring and support functions that consume large amounts of personnel time in these fields but do not require special professional training. Other retired persons with time to fill and a desire to fill it usefully have freed full-time staff from routine indirect tasks, and still others with years of professional experience and/or extensive community contacts have provided valuable expert consultation and assistance. Where older persons have been used in mental health-related services, they have been found to be important and dependable additions to meeting human resource requirements.

Whether one attempts to create formal paid work opportunities, formal volunteer roles, or increased opportunities to contribute within one's network of family, friends, and neighbors, the basic benefits are the same. Not only are more human resources made available to address mental health needs but more persons benefit from the bolstering of self-esteem that comes from helping others—in itself a "mental health service." Assistance is made available in a greater variety of forms, increasing the chances that a given individual will find help that meshes with his or her own cultural and personal perspectives. And the mental health system is enriched through more egalitarian contacts with persons outside the professional elite.

Most important, utilization of older persons as resources in the mental health system represents a strategy of *empowerment* (Solomon, 1977). The elderly are in many ways an oppressed group in that they face difficulties that are a direct product of the attitudes and responses of the dominant society toward them. One does not cease to be capable of contributing to one's community at the age of 65, but rather the 65-year-old must cope with the effects of being defined into idleness by others. The appropriate intervention in such a situation is not to wait until the inevitable depression sets in and then offer psychotherapy. Much more helpful and less victim blaming is an approach which returns to the older person control over the allocation of his or her time and energy between instrumental and expressive activities. The mental health system can be helpful to many older persons by facilitating their continued functioning as normal productive citizens and by standing in opposition to societal policies which turn such persons into mental health clients. In the words of the President's Commission (1978):

> Mental health services cannot adequately respond to the needs of the citizens of this country unless those involved in the planning, organization, and delivery of those services fully recognize the harmful effect that a variety of social, environmental, physical, psychological, and biological factors can have on the ability of individuals to function in society, develop a sense of their own worth, and maintain a strong and purposeful self-image (Vol. I, p. 9).

For older persons, being barred from opportunities for productive, other-directed activity is a major factor that must be addressed. The use of older workers in mental health endeavors is not a new idea. Many programs throughout the United States and Europe have recognized and utilized the time and talents of the elderly in many different ways. Older persons have advised, counseled, assisted, and provided support and companionship to other aged persons, children, retarded persons, hospitalized mental patients, the home-bound and handicapped, and harried parents. They have gathered data for planning, mobilized community support, reorganized files, provided clerical assistance, answered telephones, run errands, raised funds, and made policy decisions. Probably every activity that takes place within the mental health system has been provided by an older person at some time in some place. Many programs have attempted to systematically recruit older workers and volunteers and have, through experience, gained considerable understanding of the requirements and the costs and advantages of such undertakings. But the bulk of these efforts have remained isolated and have had little opportunity to benefit from the successes and failures of colleagues in other isolated projects.

It is the purpose of this book to make a first step toward rectifying the situation by

1. Drawing attention to the importance of older workers in the mental health system both as a valuable addition to the system itself and as a critical primary prevention approach to maintaining mental health among the elderly,
2. Indicating the range and depth of experience that exists in this area in the hopes that more comprehensive efforts to consolidate and communicate this knowledge will be generated, and
3. Enumerating and clarifying the major issues that are involved in such efforts so that the extent of understanding of each can be assessed and future examinations can be targeted on the most critical and least understood issues.

Toward those ends, contributions describing, analyzing, and evaluating a number of existing programs are presented. Most of these utilize older workers and/or volunteers in roles that attempt to link potential clients to existing professional services or to make such services more easily accessible. In addition, older persons are seen providing direct services ranging from counseling to concrete assistance and developing program support within the community at large. Experiences from three countries (United States, Israel, and Canada) are included as well as programs in differing cultural communities within the United States.

Part II presents four different program models that are suggestive, though by no means inclusive, of the diverse roles in which older workers/volunteers are currently found in mental health and health network. Some of the strengths and limitations of each model are suggested.

First, Diamond, Brown, and Estes describe a comprehensive geriatric program within a community mental health center that incorporates older persons as resources in a variety of ways. Elderly from the community have been involved in the planning process, older workers fill positions such as case aides and drivers, and older volunteers provide a wide range of direct and supportive services. The assignment of volunteer tasks is approached explicitly as a preventive therapeutic service to elderly clients. Also, extensive use of older volunteers allows for program expansion well beyond the constraints of funding. The latter is no small contribution for, as this chapter makes clear, considerable budgetary ingenuity is required to piece together a truly comprehensive mental health program from the funding sources that are available.

Next, the use of retired persons as voluntary workers in an Israeli national program is presented by Blumensohn. In spite of whatever cultural differences may exist, the tasks performed by older volunteers are strikingly similar to those encountered in American programs. It is notable that this volunteer force consists entirely of retired professionals with backgrounds relevant to the services they are to provide. Thus, the *existing* expertise of aged persons is being drawn on to meet the needs of the public sector.

Schapiro reports on an unusual effort in which older workers provided personalized rehabilitation services to deinstitutionalized adult retardates. This type of support service is typical of those the President's Commission indicated to be critical but generally lacking. In this chapter, we have a clear illustration of the value of older workers who have the time and patience to provide labor-intensive, highly individualized services. Again, the expected benefits to the workers were part of the design.

Finally, in the chapter by Tristan and Bakke, we expand our consideration to the broader field of health—specifically maternal and

child services, where health and mental health are especially insepar-
able. Further, since this project existed in a predominantly Mexican-
American community, we are reminded that "old age" is partially
defined by cultural realities and expectations. Tristan and Bakke discuss
the importance of a group of the community's designated elders in
generating understanding of and support for the services being made
available. Here we see older volunteers providing critical links between
the organization and the community rather than focusing solely on
direct services to single individuals.

Part III gives closer attention to the benefits, costs, and limitations
of utilizing older workers and/or volunteers in mental health programs.
Several viewpoints are presented and the levels of consideration touch
on specific operational and therapeutic issues as well as global
evaluations.

McCaslin and Wilson begin by drawing on their experience in
developing a comprehensive geriatric mental health program in Texas
to discuss the overall costs and benefits of including older workers on
the staff. Race and sex as well as age are identified as relevant worker
characteristics. They take the position that the addition of older
workers makes for notable changes both in supervisory tasks and in
program outputs and that staff should accept the total situation as
different rather than focusing on only costs or benefits.

A brief chapter by Trelease explores in greater detail one of the
issues older workers may bring to their task—the need to accept
themselves as aging persons and at the same time reject the stereotype
of "the useless old" through their own activity. Three cases are used to
indicate the various ways individual workers attempt to resolve this
dilemma and the implications are discussed.

Next, Kowalski provides an in-depth description of a single,
federally funded older-volunteers program—one of several which
might be drawn on in developing the type of system discussed by
Diamond et al. in part II. Focusing on the experience of Rhode Island's
Senior Companion Program and drawing from the evaluative statements of its older workers, Kowalski not only details the diverse
functions of the companions and the benefits they themselves receive,
but also conveys a feeling for the elderly involved in this project and
their attitudes toward their activities. What emerges is a strong
argument for the therapeutic value of being enabled to help others.

Finally, Bristowe describes a Canadian program which, again,
bears a striking resemblance to those included from the United States
and Israel. In a thoughtful discussion of the operation of such programs,

she raises the possibility of negative secondary outcomes for older workers serving even older and frailer elderly. The position taken is that it may be more beneficial to both designated helper and client to cross-match age and problem groups when designing paraprofessional systems.

Part IV moves to a more general level of discussion and places the experiences included in the first two sections in the context of a review of the relevant literature. Consideration is given to existing opinions and evidence in relation to (1) the contributions that mental health programs employing older persons make to the older workers/volunteers themselves, (2) the unique contributions that older workers and volunteers can make to mental health programs, (3) unresolved operational issues that are important to the efficiency and effectiveness of such programs and to their usefulness to both clients and workers, (4) the value of normalization and empowerment strategies that stress the development of needed roles for older persons as opposed to traditional treatment approaches, and (5) the need for evaluative research on older worker/volunteer programs. It is the aim of this section to clarify the state of the art so that priorities may be better developed for future efforts.

In general, the chapters that follow contain varying combinations of program description and issue analysis. It is hoped that in this way the perceptions of older workers and volunteers themselves will be a part of the discussion, as well as those of researchers and practitioners. It is our contention that programs employing older workers will be optimally effective if they are viewed as a partnership between young and old, professional and lay person, formed to enhance the mental health of all people.

References

Austin, M. J. *Professionals and Paraprofessionals.* New York: Human Sciences Press, 1978.

Barker, R. L., and Briggs, T. L. *Differential Use of Social Work Manpower.* New York: National Association of Social Workers, 1968.

Caplan, G., and Killilea, M. (eds.). *Support Systems and Mutual Help: Multidisciplinary Explorations.* New York: Grune and Stratton, 1976.

Cohen, R. *New Careers Grows Older: A Perspective on the Paraprofessional Experience, 1965–1975.* Baltimore: Johns Hopkins Press, 1976.

Collins, A. H., and Pancoast, D. L. *Natural Helping Networks: A Strategy for Prevention.* Washington, D.C.: National Association of Social Workers (no date).

Comfort, A. Age prejudice in America. In F. Riessman (ed.), *Older Persons: Unused Resources for Unmet Needs.* Beverly Hills: Sage, 1977.

Department of Health, Education and Welfare. *Overview Study of Employment of Paraprofessionals.* Research Report No. 3' Washington, D.C., 1974.

Epstein, L. Differential use of staff: A method to expand social services. *Social Work,* 1962, 7, 66–72.

Friedmann, E. A., and Havighurst, R. J. *The Meaning of Work and Retirement.* Chicago: University of Chicago Press, 1954.

Gaitz, C. M. (ed.). *Aging and the Brain.* New York: Plenum Press, 1972.

Gershon, M., and Biller, H. B. *The Other Helpers: Paraprofessionals and Nonprofessionals in Mental Health.* Lexington: Lexington Books, 1977.

Grosser, C., Henry, W. E., and Kelly, J. G. *Nonprofessionals in the Human Services.* San Franciso: Jossey-Bass, 1969.

Harris, L., and Associates, Inc. *The Myth and Reality of Aging in America.* Washington, D.C.: National Council on the Aging, 1975.

Heyman, M. M. Criteria for the allocation of cases according to levels of staff skill. *Social Casework,* 1966, 47, 325–331.

Kahn, R. L., Zarit, S. H., Hilbert, H. M., and Niederehe, G. Memory complaint and impairment in the aged. *Archives of General Psychiatry,* 1975, 32, 1569–1573.

Kent, D. P., Hirsch, C., and Barg, S. K. Indigenous workers as a crucial link in the total support system for low-income minority group aged: A report of an innovative field technique in survey research. *International Journal of Aging and Human Development,* 1971, 2, 189–196.

President's Commission on Mental Health. *Report to the President,* Vols. I–IV. Washington, D.C.: U.S. Gov. Printing Office, 1978.

Richan, W. C. A theoretical scheme for determining roles of professional and nonprofessional personnel. *Social Work,* 1961, 6, 22–28.

Richan, W. C. (ed.). *Human Services and Social Work Responsibility.* New York: National Association of Social Workers, 1969.

Richan, W. C. Indigenous paraprofessional staff. In Kaslow and Associates (eds.), *Issues in Human Services.* San Francisco: Jossey-Bass, 1972.

Sarason, S. B., and Lorentz, E. *The Challenge of the Resource Exchange Network.* San Francisco: Jossey-Bass, 1979.

Solomon, B. B. *Black Empowerment: Social Work in Oppressed Communities.* New York: Columbia University Press, 1977.

Varner, R. V. Clinical assessment, expectations, and total management of organic brain syndromes in the elderly. *Southern Medicine,* 1976, Oct. 23–28.

Varner, R. V., and Calvert, W. R. Psychological assessment of the aged: A differential model for diagnosis. *Journal of the American Geriatric Society,* 1974, *22,* 273–277.

Weed, V., and Denham, W. H. Toward more effective use of the nonprofessional worker: A recent experiment. *Social Work,* 1961, *6,* 29–36.

Part II
A Program Sampler

2

Older Case Aides and Volunteers in a Community Mental Health Center's Program for the Aging

Herbert Diamond
George A. Brown
Ernestine Estes

The Community Mental Health Centers' Act of 1963 (Public Law 88-164) was amended only in 1975 (Public Law 94-63) to require services for the elderly. Even though the Community Mental Health Center (CMHC) program was designed as an innovative, community-based system of services that would respond to local mental health needs, with few exceptions the thrust of program development has largely bypassed the elderly. As recently as the late 1970s, only 8 of over 600 federally funded CMHCs had developed significant, specialized services for this still largely underserved population (personal communication).

One of these centers is the West Philadelphia Community Mental Health Consortium, Inc., a decentralized, comprehensive CMHC that has developed a multifaceted program for its aging population in southwest Philadelphia (Santore and Diamond, 1974). This specialized program was pursued collaboratively with a group of clergy in the community who were particularly interested in serving their aging parishioners, even though federal mandates emphasized other program priorities.

The legislation of 1963 and amendments of 1965 (Public Law 89-105) required five basic services: inpatient, outpatient, partial hospitalization, emergency services, and consultation and education. The Commonwealth of Pennsylvania's own legislation of 1966 (Mental

Health and Mental Retardation Act) added some optional services including diagnostic evaluation, pre- and aftercare, rehabilitation, staff training, and program evaluation. Special services for specific age groups such as children and the elderly became major federal requirements in 1975 when P.L. 94-63 added 7 program areas to the original 5. However, because of funding limitations and programmatic constraints, CMHCs nationally have generally been unable to develop all 12 services, and as a result, programs for special age and disability groups have largely remained quietly cooling or simmering on back burners. These difficulties were reflected in the Mental Health Systems Act (P.L. 96-536), which reduced the number of required services but supported "new initiatives" responsive to locally identified special needs. Unfortunately, the repeal of the Mental Health Systems Act by the Administration's Omnibus Budget Reconciliation Act of 1981 further jeopardizes funding for the mentally disabled elderly. It is increasingly clear that comprehensive CMHC programs for the aging will continue to be developed at a very slow rate and to require the identification and tapping of non-CMHC funding streams. However, on the positive side of the balance sheet is the implementation by the Joint Commission on Accreditation of Hospitals (JCAH) of its accreditation program for community mental health service programs (Principles for Accreditation, 1966). JCAH now requires some responsiveness by CMHCs to the needs of four identified age groups, including the elderly, in order for a center to become accredited.

However, in spite of funding inadequacies, institutional barriers, and professional apathy, it is possible for CMHCs to respond to the multiple needs of the aging, and crucial participants in this effort are the elderly themselves. This chapter will discuss one of the center's programs and the varied roles and contributions of the elderly themselves that have helped make it work.

The West Philadelphia Community Mental Health Consortium, Inc.

The West Philadelphia Community Mental Health Consortium is a comprehensive community mental health and mental retardation center that is now in its 14th year of developing decentralized services in southwest Philadelphia. It is an affiliation within the community of four hospitals, the West Philadelphia Corporation, a planning agency, the University of Pennsylvania and its Department of Psychiatry, the Philadelphia Child Guidance Clinic, the Philadelphia College of Osteopathic Medicine, and the Elwyn Institute. Since 1969 equal numbers of institutional and community members have been represented on the board of directors and its committees. It serves a catchment area (CA 3) of 22 square miles containing a population of 203,000.

The agency's strength lies in its responsiveness to its community's mental health concerns and needs. It has reached out to its many "subcommunities" and highly diversified populations through a network of neighborhood counseling centers. In addition, it provides psychiatric inpatient care, emergency and partial hospitalization services, aftercare, children's services, consultation and education, services for the mentally retarded, drug and alcholism programs, counseling for women in transition, and an older adult program.

The 1970 decennial census showed that the 65-and-over population represented 10 percent of the catchment area's total population of 202,871. During the year July 1, 1971 to June 30, 1972, elderly patients composed only 3.7 percent of total registrations. However, by the year July 1, 1975 through June 30, 1976, this figure had increased to 6.6 percent. It increased further to 7.9 percent in FY 80–81, and a goal of 10 percent is projected. Although the elderly remained underrepresented in the total patient population, the significant increase of elderly actively served by the CMHC reflected both the special effort made to reach them and the expanding influence of the agency's older adult programs. Currently, just under 300 patients 65 and over are being seen jointly in a counseling center and in older adult services regarding mental health, drugs, or alcohol problems. These varied outpatient services, therefore, are being provided in both supportive and natural environments and are aimed at stabilization, growth, and sustenance goals (Principles for Accreditation, 1966).

The Older Adult Project

Through the outreach activities of one counseling center (southwest) in early 1970, staff became aware of a newly established organization of Protestant churches, called Community Celebration, whose clergy was particularly concerned about the older in their parishes. Stimulated by the potential of a joint undertaking, the agency collaborated in planning for an initial demonstration project to attempt to better serve the mental health needs of the community's older residents. It was anticipated that such an actively outreaching program could help to identify and alleviate some of the problems of older persons and enhance some aspects of their day-to-day living.

Coincidentally, at this time the University of Pennsylvania School of Medicine's Department of Community Medicine was developing a gerontology project and had a small budgetary surplus. With state approval, a small grant from those funds was approved for a 10-week pilot project. The main objectives of the Older Adult Project were to

1. Provide outreach, support, information, referral, and direct casework assistance to the elderly in areas of medical, financial, mental health, recreation, and home help services
2. Train selected older local residents to use their talents and interest in working with the elderly
3. Provide a visible symbol of concern for the aged
4. Act as an advocacy link between resources and older people, and
5. Document need and stimulate the creation of new and preventive services (Santore and Diamond, 1974)

A uniquely important aspect of the project's design involved the recruitment of eight case aids who were all over 60 years of age and who lived in the community to be served. They were paid $2.20 an hour for a 20-hour work week for the duration of the 10-week pilot. Care was taken by the aides themselves to limit this additional income so that it did not interfere with their Social Security benefits. Their training included presentations on aging, senility, interviewing, casework, helping relationships, terminal illness, welfare, Medicare, and Social Security.

The success of this initial effort, which developed a caseload of over 150 and mobilized both interest and expectations in the community prompted the agency to identify and allocate funds for its continuation. A staff report summarized and evaluated the initial project as follows:

> This project has provided direct services to older adults and has also served as a tool by which to assess the community's needs and services in regard to the aged. Most older adults receive care of some sort. They attend medical clinics, live in public housing, receive welfare, are seen at a

counseling center or are a concern to neighbors, family or their church. However, this nonsystem of concern lacks continuity and focus. People get lost in the cracks. By providing information and referral, personal care of individuals becomes more complete. A vital linkage is established between the various community agencies. By working with churches, nursing homes, health agencies, doctors, clinics, social service staffs, welfare departments and the community mental health centers a cooperative and more comprehensive system of care begins to emergy. . . .

This project has utilized the services of eight local older adult persons (age sixty and over) who use their appreciation and concern for the situation of other persons to assist in cases where support is needed. This includes such things as making home visits, determining the needs of the people, contacting appropriate resources to meet the needs, providing transportation, establishing and continuing a supportive relationship, record keeping, cheering the lonely, and case finding. . . . These workers bring with them understanding, rapport, natural warmth and spontaneity. The project, concomitantly, provides an opportunity for meaningful use of the time and talents of the eight employed older adults. . . .

This program has been enthusiastically received by the individuals concerned and the community, and has been an invaluable tool in reaching the traditionally "hard to reach" older adults. With a minimum of this kind of support, many have been able to retain their independence and remain in their own homes. Based on our experience, we have found that not only has our service been a critically needed one, but it has uncovered a volume of unmet needs of the older adult, which indicates the need for an expansion of services of this program, as well as initiating similar programs in other parts of our catchment area (Townsend, 1972).

In the following year the caseload was increased, transportation services were initiated, a drop-in center was created, and older persons in the area became better organized to develop other services and activities. From that tentative beginning 10½ years ago and nurtured by the enthusiastic collaboration of the church group, CMHC, staff, elderly in the community, the State of Pennsylvania, the Philadelphia Corporation for Aging (PCA), and the local funding authority, the program has steadily grown to include a comprehensive range of services. The staff is now composed of about 45 persons, 20 percent of whom are over the age of 60. The program is funded by the Philadelphia Corporation for Aging, which provides 75 percent of the budget, and the Philadelphia County Office of Mental Health/Mental Retardation, which provides a 25 percent cash match.

Nutritional services are provided to 310 individuals on a daily basis through a hot noontime meal, with an additional 100 meals delivered to homebound individuals. Since mobility is essential for day-to-day living and since many are unable to move around safely and adequately, transportation is provided for travel back and forth to the centers, for clinic and medical appointments, for shopping and banking trips. Four of the program's six drivers are older persons.

Social services are managed by social workers and elderly case aides. This staff is responsible for the social service needs of center participants, homebound clients, and community residents. The social workers are also responsible for assessing client needs for home-delivered services and arranging for their provision. Information and referral are an integral part of these services and are offered to the entire older adult community.

Until January 1979, the staff nurse functioned as health coordinator and was involved in a wide range of activities. She personally did basic health screenings and blood pressure monitoring for both center and homebound clients. In addition, she developed and scheduled health educational programs, worked closely with family physicians, and scheduled regular clinic appointments. Through the efforts of the staff nurse a blood bank program was organized.

Socialization and recreation activities occur daily at each of the centers. The senior citizens are actively involved in physical exercise programs, trips, educational programs, arts and crafts, drama, and bazaars. Many of the designated activities were initiated by the participants themselves.

Other services include outreach through newspapers, radio, and television publicity, telephone reassurance, chore services, and a food cooperative from which collective purchases may be made at reduced cost. A relationship with a rehabilitation institute has been established so that a lip-reading course can be given to assist some of the hard-of-hearing participants.

One of the program's largest services is the volunteer service provided by 120 older volunteers. Their activities includes serving lunch, typing, keeping records, conducting programs, and making friendly visits. These services, which are preventive in nature, currently serve about 1,400 individuals who are actively involved with the program.

Related Community Services

A foundation grant has provided initial funding for a Geriatric Day Hospital that was initially located in one of the agency's member hospitals, but now operates in one of the center's own facilities. This program is geared to disabled elderly who have psychiatric problems associated with their physical illnesses. Medical services are provided by a general physician and, as needed, by local hospitals and their clinics. Nursing, social service, physical and speech therapy, recreational therapy, and other supports are built into this service. Clients receive transportation to and from the program. Financial support also comes from Medicaid reimbursement, and efforts are under way to qualify for Medicare as well. The day hospital serves 17–20 persons daily and is growing rapidly. A grant of $150,000 was awarded by Philadelphia's Community Development Office to renovate space in a building for the program.

The In-Home Service Program and Domiciliary Care are two programs that also are administrated by the local area agency on aging (PCA). They are, however, an integral part of the larger service system. The Older Adult Service administrative office houses the in-home service coordinators and a part-time secretary. They make assessments and reassessments from the consortium's social service staff referrals and broker the homemaker service from a number of private home health agencies. Domiciliary care is also a slowly growing part of PCA's program. The Older Adult Service is linked into the program by staff referral and follow-up.

The funding for all of these services varies somewhat from year to year. The multipurpose senior centers combine Title IV of the Older Americans Act, Title XX of the Social Security Act, state-appropriated funds, and the 25 percent county match. As noted, the Geriatric Day Hospital has been funded initially by a private foundation and is currently funded by Medicaid. A recent report summarizes funding sources for programs for the elderly (Wilson and Simson, 1980).

The Senior Citizen as Case Aide

Very little of this achievement would have been possible without the enthusiastic and productive participation of the community's older residents, particularly the case aids and volunteers. A report on the project cited earlier (Santore and Diamond, 1974) described the following aspects of the case aide experience and role:

> The project successfully utilized the services of the older case aides, who very effectively used their energy, concerns, and skills in helping ways, cheering those who were lonely, reaching many isolated individuals

traditionally hard to reach, and uncovering a volume of unmet needs. At the same time this program provided the aides with an opportunity for meaningful use of their own time and talents. . . .

The experience of the initial demonstration project did identify difficulties encountered in utilizing older workers as case aides.

Problems occasionally occurred when aides played favorites, producing an imbalance of service to others. There were other "counter-transference" difficulties when, through overidentification, some aides took client problems home with them, upsetting their own equanimity. Some anxiety and conflict occurred in response to change in work schedules, and a few aides tended to exhaust themselves without adequate regard for their own physical and emotional limitations. Personal and health problems forced the resignation of two of the original staff, and some consideration has been given to lowering the age limit to fifty-five.

In spite of these problems, the use of older workers was seen as a valuable addition to the program. The impact of their presence both on the total community and on the program has been profound. With supervision this group of previously untrained individuals became effective in the delivery of services to other older persons. Based on this success, the program subsequently began to expand its services through the use of elderly persons in a variety of volunteer roles.

The Senior Citizen as Volunteer

Today there are 120 persons aged 60 years and older who serve as volunteers in the older adult programs of the consortium. The volunteers are individuals who are eligible to receive the services offered by the center and in fact are chosen from program participants to assist staff in service delivery. When an older person enters the center, the voluntary program is explained and the visitor is given the opportunity to volunteer. Many individuals come to the program with an expectation of functioning as volunteers. Individuals usually volunteer for a specific task and for one day or a portion of a day may be a volunteer and at another time a participant.

Volunteers are identifiable at the center by the special badge they wear. In addition, names of active volunteers for the day are posted on the bulletin board. They meet monthly to discuss issues common to volunteers, and periodically staff plan volunteer recognition activities. An annual testimonial luncheon thanks them with plaques or certificates.

These older volunteers bring with them experience of living and familiarity with the community as well as specific knowledge from their life's vocation. They are involved in a wide variety of activities and their participation broadens the scope of the program. They help to set up the noontime meal and clean up afterward, run special groups such as sewing, crafts, and art, and assume responsibility for organizing and conducting bazaars and other fundraising activities. Homebound participants can expect a friendly visit from a volunteer who has similar interests and concerns. Many act as chaperones for medical appointments while others are involved in assisting with minor home repairs. The older adult center is an extremely active place, and it commonly impresses visitors with its purposeful activity, involvements, and clearly expressed concern for its clients.

The older volunteers contribute a unique enthusiasm to the center's environment as they radiate exuberance, commitment, energy, and a desire to do whatever is necessary to keep things moving. Their generation is a work-oriented one, and this is reflected in their strong commitment to keep busy. For many of them employment was the focal point of their lives, and the experience of retirement, if this were to mean inactivity, would be devastating. They are no longer welcome in the world of employment, but they are welcomed and valued at their senior citizen center. This activity helps them to continue viewing themselves as valued and useful individuals.

There are both pluses and minuses to using elderly participants as volunteers. Older persons usually have more time to give and offer it freely and willingly while making few demands for rewards. They bring a wide range of knowledge and experience, which adds color and dimension to the program, and they can be depended on to carry out predetermined tasks and to assume additional ones should the need arise. On the other hand, their need for activity and their over-exuberance put a unique kind of responsibility and pressure on staff to be well organized and in control of the program while coordinating the needs of all the participants, both volunteers and nonvolunteers.

Staff willingly delegate authority to the volunteers to perform certain tasks. There are many volunteers who were experts in their fields and accustomed to functioning in positions of authority. This capability can be an important asset in making it possible for volunteers to plan independently for and to teach a group of their peers. Such delegated authority ends once the designated activity is completed. However, sometimes volunteers have difficulty making the transition from leader to follower and may alienate other participants or the volunteer leader of the next activity by attempting to control that activity also. Because of close working relationships with staff, some volunteers begin to feel superior to nonvolunteer participants and to assume staff functions. In spite of such problems, it is clear that an older adult program is strengthened by the contributions of the older volunteers.

Future Trends

The Older Adult Project benefited the CMHC by helping it to develop a positive community image. The question of image is a significant factor as the stigma of receiving care for a mental condition will likely be prevalent among a large segment of the senior citizen population. Many senior citizens come from a generation of Americans who place value on self-reliance and rugged individualism. Seeking help of any nature may be adverse to their basic values. Despite this, the increased use of the CMHC can likely be attributed to the destigmatizing of mental health (preventive services) as characterized by the linkage of multipurpose senior centers with CMHCs, thereby making mental health services more palatable. The case aides also did much to generate patients for both counseling and senior centers through their outreach efforts, and the older adults made excellent workers available to the CMHC at modest cost. Because the senior case aides were so effective, their role expanded along with the program.

The long-range goal of the Older Adult Service remains that of becoming a primary social service, health, and mental health delivery system for the elderly in southwest Philadelphia. A central issue that needs to be emphasized targets on the role of the older adult worker/ volunteer in the system. The Older Adult Service is strengthened by its philosophy that older persons are capable of productive work and that they should be encouraged to be an active part of the program in order to enhance consumer linkages as well as their own socialization, functionality, and self-esteem.

The program will continue to utilize older workers as volunteers, professional workers, and case aides. In planning for the future, two new areas are seen for the utilization of the older worker. First, the problem of substance abuse among the elderly is increasingly evident. Alcoholism and drug dependence are disabling large numbers of older adults. In order to respond to this need, plans are under way to utilize older workers and volunteers in an outreach program to locate elderly substance abusers and to help them utilize both the mental health and alcoholism and drug services of the CMHC. If properly trained, older workers seem to be ideally suited to relate to this essentially withdrawn and hard-to-reach population.

In addition, the agency intends to facilitate the use of older employees in the community's work force. Many older workers are forced out of jobs and need and want to continue working because of either financial reasons or interest in the activity itself. Current plans include the development of a job bank program which will identify and create part-time jobs for the elderly in area businesses and set up small businesses for older people in ways that will avoid union conflict. These programs will be devloped by the older adults themselves as funding is obtained.

Older workers have played a crucial role in the development of the Consortium's Older Adult Service as senior case aides and as volunteers. Without their skill, energy, and commitment, such complex services simply could not have been delivered. It is hoped that other community agencies can benefit from these experiences, which indicate that funds for programs for the aging can be identified and mobilized, that bureaucratic barriers can be bypassed, and that the political power of the elderly can be harnessed to support programs for them and in which they actively participate.

References

Mental Health and Mental Retardation Act of 1966, 1966 Special Sess. No. 3, October 20, P.L. 96. Commonwealth of Pennsylvania.

Personal communication from the Office of Aging, ADAMHA.

Principles for Accreditation of Community Mental Health Service Programs. Joint Commission on Accreditation of Hospitals, 1966.

Santore, A. F., and Diamond, H. The role of a community mental health center in developing services to the aging: The Older Adult Project. *The Gerontologist*, 1974, *14*, 201–206.

Townsend, E. A *Status Report of the Older Adult Project.* August 18, 1972.
Wilson, L. B., and Simson, S. Community mental health centers and the elderly: A time for expansion of planning, research, and demonstration projects. *Community Mental Health Journal,* 1980, *16*, 276–282.

3

Retired People Counsel the Aged: The National Insurance Institute of Israel, Counseling Centers for Senior Citizens

Leo Blumensohn

Counseling Centers for Senior Citizens

When the State of Israel was established in 1948, it had on the average a young population. Thus, it is only in recent years that the country has begun to face the problems of old age and of aging. The founding generation that built the state was largely unaware of the problems of old age in those early years, but upon reaching retirement age they came to realize that they had failed to set up suitable institutions that could meet the needs of an ever-growing elderly population. Those institutions that have been established over the years, such as "golden age clubs" and old-age homes, cater to only a very small number of pensioners and many retired persons have been at a loss as to whom and where to turn for assistance with regard to their problems.

The idea of establishing counseling centers arose from the need and desire to reach a large proportion of the older population. It was natural that these counseling centers be created within the framework of the National Insurance Institute to which every older person must

The National Insurance Institute is the public agency which administers Israel's national social security system. Its branches include old age and survivor's, disability, work injury, maternity, children, unemployment, rights of workers in bankruptcy or corporate dissolution, and reserve service. The institute also administers the alimony law, the benefit payments for persons with limited mobility, equity grants, the victims of hostile action law, and the rights of volunteers law.

eventually apply personally in order to submit his or her claim for an old age pension. This was thought to be an ideal opportunity with which to inform older persons of the services available and to allow for discussion of their problems at leisure, in a calm and intimate atmosphere with a friendly counselor. The counselors, themselves pensioners, would be professionals with extensive experience in the field. Thus they would inspire confidence professionally but, above all, through readiness to lend a friendly ear.

In 1972 the first counseling centers were opened as experimental models—one in Ramat Gan, the other in Jerusalem. By 1977, 6 such regional centers as well as 18 secondary centers were in operation at the branch offices of the National Insurance Institute. Within the next three years additional counseling centers were established at all branches of the Institute.

All counselors were to be volunteer pensioners whose education was commensurate with their task. They were to be either experienced in social and public work (e.g., social workers, public health nurses) or trained in specific professions (e.g., experts on occupation and pension funds, professionals in the legal field, businesspersons). Every counseling center was to be managed by a paid professional worker—either a social worker, a psychologist, or a sociologist—who would work together with the volunteer counselors, forming a congenial, cooperative staff.

The principal objective of these centers was to be the improvement of delivery of existing services and the formation of new services for the benefit of the older population. Toward that end, counseling was not seen as terminating merely with "good counsels." It should aim to help the pensioner either through short-term assistance by the counselor or by referral to the proper authorities. In all instances, cases were to be closely followed up.

Initiative to Develop Additional Services

Several months after the first counseling centers were opened it was found that veteran pensioners who had been receiving old age and survivors' pensions for years failed to come to the centers. It was concluded that volunteers must be trained to work in the neighborhood and in old age centers in order to reach these veteran pensioners who might not be aware of their rights. Work in the neighborhood indicated a need for home visits, especially among senior citizens confined to their homes. The first visit was mainly devoted to informing the pensioners of their rights and was often followed by other visits, usually initiated by the volunteer, upon discovering difficult and complex personal problems besetting the homebound person. Subsequent to these activities, it was deemed necessary to organize subgroups of volunteers, mainly from the neighborhood, who receive professional guidance both from the supervisor of the center and from other professional workers. More and more home visits were promoted and the project was encouraged and supported by the local authorities.

Aims of the Program

The following were established as the primary aims of every counseling center:

1. To develop the center as a place to which older persons feel they can come for information, guidance, and advice. More important, however, it should be a place where older people feel they can be at ease, where problems can be discussed in a comfortable and intimate atmosphere, and where clients are sure to find a sympathetic ear.

2. To form groups of volunteer pensioners from persons in the liberal professions or whose education is commensurate with the necessary tasks, who are ready to serve as counselors and guides to other members of the older population. It is assumed that a pensioner with many years of experience in a helping profession is most suitable to advise other pensioners. Such persons are closely acquainted with problems of new pensioners because they have likely also had to cope with them. At the same time, the work itself and the satisfaction of being of help to other older people may provide an opportunity for volunteers to realize their own aspirations to remain active and do challenging work.

3. To improve existing services and their delivery and to develop new services.

Current Areas of Service

Figure 1 shows the various services provided through the Counseling Program for Senior Citizens and their relation to other public services. Those services include the following:

1. Counseling for personal and social matters. Counselors deal with all personal problems arising from retirement from work, relations between the older couple, relations between parents and children, economic and social problems, and, above all, problems of loneliness. Every pensioner coming to the counseling center has the opportunity to discuss his or her problems at length and at ease and to return for further advice. Should the need arise, the pensioner is referred to other services. In such cases, the volunteer counselor coordinates necessary meetings with the relevant organizations.

   Special attention is accorded to newly widowed older (55+) women who submit claims to the National Insurance Institute for Survivors' Allowance. Such widows are personally invited to the Counseling Centers for Senior Citizens for an introductory meeting. Support for widows may be either on an individual basis or within a group framework. Weekly meetings are held over an extended period with voluntary social workers advising and counseling the groups. Counseling focuses not only on alleviating the pain inherent in the loss of a spouse and resultant loneliness, but also deals with the adjustment to a new social status.

2. Take up rights. Advice is provided regarding rights and benefits about which the pensioner is ignorant, whether these be pension rights through the National Insurance Institute or pensions or other benefits provided by various governmental bodies, the municipality, and the General Labor Federation. In order to reach persons who are not aware of these rights, a reaching-out program is maintained whereby volunteers visit homes, clubs frequented by the aged, synagogues, and even park benches in order to inform potential clients of available services and to examine whether they have indeed taken advantage of their rights.

3. Legal advice. The pensioner has access to professional legal advice (from a volunteer lawyer) regarding problems such as the transfer of property and inheritance, change of age (the age

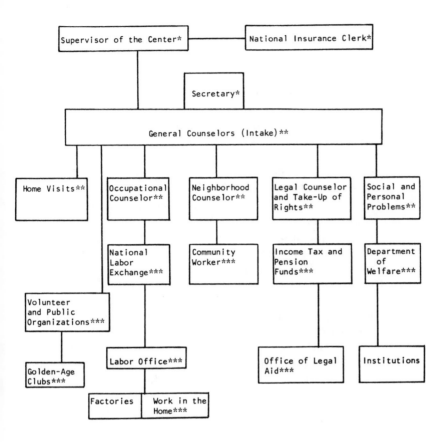

| Supervisor of the Center* | National Insurance Clerk* |

Secretary*

General Counselors (Intake)**

| Home Visits** | Occupational Counselor** | Neighborhood Counselor** | Legal Counselor and Take-Up of Rights** | Social and Personal Problems** |

| National Labor Exchange*** | Community Worker*** | Income Tax and Pension Funds*** | Department of Welfare*** |

Volunteer and Public Organizations***

| Golden-Age Clubs*** | Labor Office*** | Office of Legal Aid*** | Institutions |

| Factories | Work in the Home*** |

*   Employees of the National Insurance Institute
**   Volunteers
***   National and Public Services

FIGURE 1. Counseling Program for Senior Citizens and Its Relation to Other Public Services

having been erroneously registered on the identification card due to the special conditions prevalent at the time of immigration to Israel), and rental disputes (the fine points of the rental protection law).

4. Work and occupation. The pensioner is given advice and concrete assistance in obtaining full or part-time work through individual placement. Attempts are also made to bring work to community centers within the neighborhood for those in need of additional income who cannot travel to work outside their immediate neighborhood (in coordination with the national occupational services of the Ministry of Labor).

The volunteer occupational counselors at the counseling centers are constantly in touch with all types of factories, workshops, institutions, and governmental agencies. After interviewing a pensioner seeking work, they direct him or her to a suitable place of employment. In special cases, and according to the demands of the labor market, the pensioner is given professional training which is carried out by the Labor Exchange. Those primarily interested in occupying their time rather than supplementing their income are directed to social centers and to "golden age clubs." There, in addition to the usual activities offered, they have access to a community worker or professional who will assist them in finding a hobby, such as sculpture, painting, or ceramics.

Newly retired persons who are capable of fulfilling a role in a volunteer capacity at the counseling centers are invited to join the program. The remainder are referred to other voluntary organizations, according to criteria based on degree of interest, area of expertise, and the capability of the pensioner in question.

5. Home visits to ill and homebound aged. A great many volunteers are engaged in the home visit program to lone and ill homebound aged. A visit usually entails a social call and the volunteer functions as a friend as well as a liaison between the homebound person and the various outside agencies with whom he or she is in contact. In actuality, most of the volunteers execute tasks over and above those which they were originally assigned, such as aid in daily shopping, bringing medicines, and accompanying the ill aged to the local health fund clinic.

A home visit takes place at least once a week, thus creating a close bond between the homebound person and the volunteer and enabling the latter to observe changes in the ill person's condition and to subsequently inform the proper agency. The home visit program maintains close coordination with all appropriate agencies within the community and in particular with the home care staff of the health insurance funds, hospitals, and welfare bureaus. Thus, the home visit program serves to complement the functions of the home care programs run by various institutions and contributes a great deal to the general welfare of the ill and homebound aged.

6. Development of contact with community services. Contact is made with all existing organizations which may potentially contribute to the improved welfare of the aged. The aim is to make these institutions sharply aware of and sensitive to the basic needs of older persons, and efforts are made to initiate necessary programs which aim to improve the life conditions of the elderly.

Training of Volunteers

Every new group of volunteers receives comprehensive training regarding the problems (psychological and physiological) of old age and aging, the social and health services available within the community and benefits provided by the National Insurance Institute and other pension funds. Training is mainly carried out through lectures, discussions, and study days. Over a period of three months the volunteers are also organized in small groups where they are taught the basics of good interviewing. Much emphasis is placed on the identification of needs and problems by developing the volunteer's sensitivity and ability to be a good listener. The volunteer also receives continuing in-service training within the framework of working groups at the centers which are supervised by professional workers. Supervision focuses mainly on day-to-day activities of volunteers at the counseling center and on the special problems they face in dealing with clients.

The team spirit fostered in each of the counseling centers contributes much to the volunteers' feeling that they are not alone and that there are others who also grapple with similar problems that are sometimes difficult and complex. The fact that no volunteer dropped out during the first five years of the program may be attributed to the supportive environment within which the counselor works.

Special Services

1. Cooperation with psychiatric clinics. The counseling center serving the Ramat Gan area maintains a direct link with the psychiatric clinic of the regional hospital and with the director of the clinic. Two volunteer psychiatric social workers under the supervision of the director of the clinic interview and classify applicants who have been referred by the counselors or home visitors, subsequently placing them in the care of the clinic if necessary. Application to the clinic is made directly rather than through the usual bureaucratic channels. It is worthy of mention that those aged referred to the psychiatric clinic also undergo general medical examinations at the geriatric ward of the hospital or, alternately, are referred to a psychiatric hospital for more intensive treatment. This service serves a dual function: on the one hand, it assists in preventive care in order to arrest possible deterioration and, on the other hand, it eliminates bureaucratic delay through direct referral to psychiatric treatment in acute cases.

2. Joint operation of a geriatric rehabilitation center. Joint programs are maintained with a neighborhood geriatric center which aim to (1) prevent mental and physical deterioration and (2) rehabilitate aged persons subsequent to mental or physical illness. The geriatric ward of a hospital supplies professional personnel to the center while the volunteers seek out and refer those aged who are in need of treatment. The volunteers also accompany mobility-impaired aged persons to the center and fulfill needed roles within the framework of the geriatric center itself. Among the functions they serve are providing aid in the actualization of rights and acting as links between various institutions and community servics and those aged who cannot perform these tasks for themselves.

3. Surveys to ascertain needs and actualization of rights. The volunteers participate in surveys which attempt to ascertain the needs and requirements as well as the actualization of rights of aged persons. Such surveys are jointly conducted with municipal authorities, primarily in distressed communities. The objectives are to resolve problems on an individual as well as on a community level. When acute cases of distress are uncovered through these surveys, the volunteers assist the older person in contacts with the authorities and community services. They also

encourage lone aged persons to join "golden age" clubs and they engage in visits to homebound aged persons who are discovered in the course of the survey.

Conclusion

Six hundred volunteers are currently working as counselors and home visitors to senior citizens. There has been no difficulty in recruiting good professional volunteers who are deeply sensitive to the needs of other senior citizens. Because the volunteers work within the framework of the National Insurance Institute, they are able to complement the administrative function of those in charge of receiving applications for pensions by relating to the personal and social aspects of retirement.

The activities of the volunteer are positively received by local and governmental institutions and they have not encountered any difficulties in their work with such agencies. In the relationships between volunteers and professional workers, the latter benefit from the reinforcement they receive from the volunteers, while the volunteers benefit from the guidance of the professional workers. Thus, relations of trust, mutual assistance, communication, and understanding are formed between the volunteers and the professional workers, a situation that can only improve the services delivered to the older population.

4

The Older Worker and the Mentally Retarded Adult

Judith Schapiro

Many facilities, programs, and services for mentally retarded adults have been characterized as dehumanizing, operating under conditions that deny both human and civil rights. The institutional philosophy which has guided service development in this area must be supplanted by viable alternative approaches (Nooe, 1975). Since advances in medical care have enabled more retarded children to survive into adulthood, the necessity of such innovation was becoming pressing. In 1974, the National Association for Retarded Children, recognizing the need to broaden its focus, changed the word "children" in its title to "citizens." This change reaffirmed the organization's primary objective as stated in its bylaws: "To promote the general welfare of the mentally retarded of *all ages* everywhere."

For the past 20 years the focus of program development for the mentally retarded has been in the area of children and young adults. Retarded children and youth who were aided by programs created in the 1950s and 1960s have grown older and require programs to meet their changing needs. Yet few programs have been developed for the aging mentally retarded (Segal, 1975). The majority of adult mentally retarded individuals are eventually admitted to institutions because their relatives who have cared for them have died (Richards, 1975). However, since deinstitutionalization has been adopted as a concept nationwide, many developmentally disabled adults have been subsequently relocated into smaller, more personal community settings such as halfway houses, foster homes, or group homes. The physical movement from a custodial setting to an at least partial self-care facility is only half of the process. There must also be a concurrent increase in the training and counseling designed to help these persons cope effectively with their new environment in order that they might be better equipped to provide personal input into their new life-styles. Planned efforts are needed to orient these individuals to the community so that they can function as independently as possible yet have continued contact points within the mental health system (Richards, 1975).

Much of the literature on aging concerns itself with the loss of social roles and its effect on self-concept. This has been characterized by Rosow (1973) as the "rolelessness of the aged." It appears that self-esteem among the aged is related to feelings of usefulness and engaging in activities which provide a link in the relationships between generations. Studies indicate that social interaction is positively associated with life satisfaction and that not only activity but contact with others is important for the preservation of personality and the absence of depression (Rynerson, 1972).

The Foster Grandparent Program was developed to utilize the time and talents of retired persons in providing individual attention to institutionalized children, many of whom were retarded. Studies by Greenleigh Associates (1966) and Boaz (1972) indicated both that foster grandparent work experience was beneficial to the life adjustment of the aging persons in the study and that there was a positive impact on the children's development resulting from foster grandparent care and association. There was a special compatibility of emotional needs among the "helpers" and "helpees" in these programs. The older workers were regarded as having the potential to enhance the adjustment and resocialization of deinstitutionalized mentally retarded into the normal community life pattern.

The Senior Advocacy Program (Schapiro and Grob, 1976), which is described below, represents an effort to build on the positive results of the Foster Grandparent Program in developing an alternative approach to meeting the service needs of older, mentally retarded adults. The model provides for attention and assistance on a one-to-one basis for the deinstitutionalized retarded aged from a trained advocate who is a senior citizen.

Goals of the Program

It was anticipated that the Senior Advocacy Program would satisfy the purpose of increasing both the adjustment and the resocialization of newly deinstitutionalized developmentally disabled adults. This enhanced normalization would be visible in increased client independence as well as in a decrease in the percentage of reinstitutionalizations. Additionally, it was anticipated that by choosing senior citizens to serve in the advocacy role, an available and empathetic population might be tapped as a human resource to further ease the implementation of national deinstitutionalization policies. It was recognized that elderly persons have often been placed in the role of receivers of attention, of services, of material objects, but have not had the self-esteem enhancing opportunity for giving of themselves, of their resources, of their emotional output (Kalson, 1976). The Senior Advocacy Program sought to establish a syntonic interface between the needs of elderly persons and older retardates newly placed in community programs.

Selection of Clients

The selection of clients in the Senior Advocacy Program was determined by the State of Virginia descriptive code on the developmentally disabled. The code refers to any developmental handicap attributable to mental retardation, cerebral palsy, epilepsy, or any other neurological impairment originating in the individual prior to the age of 18 years, ongoing since that time and predicted to continue indefinitely, and constituting a significant handicap to that person. Initially, there were 16 clients, male and female, black and white, ranging in age from 22 to 62 years. These clients were recently released from area training centers and domiciled in group homes sponsored by the local Association for Retarded Citizens. All the clients were diagnosed as moderately or severely retarded. Language and communication skills ranged from poor to good. Five of the clients were initially rated adequate in social development, two required assistance in this area, and one was in need of intense remediation. Most had potentially good work skills.

Objectives for the Client

The objectives for the client were to provide a sequential program to meet his or her individual needs. This would include 20 hours per week of supervised training for the purpose of facilitating physical, emotional, and cognitive development. It would also include within-the-community experience to expand and strengthen normalization skills. There would be training and counseling on a one-to-one basis for the purpose of developing information and skills in using community resources and achieving independence. Much of the responsibility for the aforementioned objectives rested with the senior advocates.

Selection of Senior Advocates

The selection of older persons to be used as advocates in the Senior Advocacy Program was determined by the following criteria:

1. They should be able to relate to others (warm, flexible, sympathetic).
2. They should possess adequate physical and mental health to function maximally in a helping relationship with their client.
3. They should be sensitive in anticipating a crisis.
4. They should be able to offer preventive counseling.
5. They should have the potential and willingness to learn.

The initial screening organization was an area-wide model program for senior citizens. The final selection of the advocates was jointly decided on by a team representing the initial screening group, the local Association for Retarded Citizens, and two educational consultants (professors from the local university). One consultant was a specialist in the field of mental retardation and the other a specialist in the field of gerontology.

Before entering the orientation program, the advocates were required to have a health screening, both medical and dental, to ensure that their physical health was such that they could function in a helping relationship in order to maximize the potential of their clients. Each advocate was also given a semantic differential on three concepts:

1. How I see the developmentally disabled adult
2. How I see myself
3. How I see this program

They were required to be 60 years of age or older and to be recipients or potential recipients of welfare.

Initially, there were eight older persons identified for this program. They were each 60+, ranging in age from 61 to 71 years. Their educational levels ranged from an eighth grade education to a master's degree in education. Scores on the Weschsler Adult Intelligence Scale (WAIS) ranged from 90 to 117. Health screening showed their health to range from adequate to poor, with the following medical conditions being the most prevalent: diabetes, cardiovascular disease, arthritis, and visual impairment.

Much of the responsibility for meeting the objectives set forth for the developmentally disabled clients rested with the advocates. In addition, each advocate was expected to do the following:

1. Identify the unmet needs of their clients
2. Locate or organize services pertinent to meeting those needs
3. Facilitate the resocialization and reintegration of their client into the mainstream of the community
4. Increase their client's social and physical development, and
5. Increase competency for their clients in relation to such activities as using money, shopping, and social visiting to places of interest

Many of these objectives were part of the scheduled 20 hours per week of one-to-one sessions. It was anticipated that from this close inter-action each advocate would form valid and realistic expectations regarding the physical and mental development of his or her client.

Program Support

The Area-wide Model Program, a federally funded and state-supported program for senior citizens, and the local branch of the Association for Retarded Citizens established collaborative support with the representative from the university. All agencies desired to assist the developmentally disabled adults and senior advocates in their own continued growth and development. All agencies provided input for the necessary personnel to develop training programs and supplied technical assistance for their implementation as needed. Dissemination of the information resulting from the program was an essential goal for each organization in order to encourage replication of this pilot program. The two university professors, acting as codirectors, were able to coordinate the efforts of participating agencies and establish a training program for replication.

Program Procedures

There were several preliminary criteria to be met prior to the program's inception. It was decided that the advocates should be paid for 20 hours of work per week which would be spent in one-to-one learning situations with their clients. This was thought to provide a valid test of the program's ability to increase the self-worth of the advocates in order to raise their morale, to improve work effectiveness, and to encourage a sense of commitment. Additionally, the advocates should perceive themselves to be economically reinvolved with their community-at-large. All agencies agreed to establish wages at the minimum level. A training program was designed for the advocates to facilitate their developing helping relationships with their clients. Initially, there was an eight-day in-service training program which included the following:

1. Health and nonhealth screening
2. Overview of the state's mental health system
3. An introduction to human growth and development
4. The concepts and characteristics of the developmentally disabled adult
5. Techniques for helpers in human relationships, such as attending, listening, conveying, understanding, and planning for action
6. Role playing and simulation
7. Information about human resource agencies pertinent to the developmentally disabled adult, including eligibility criteria, services available, typical client profiles, and appropriate referral techniques

The training program was also designed to leave the advocates with both the desire and the capability to continue developing their ability to be helpful to their clients. Therefore, the following were incorporated:

1. Information on pertinent state and human resource agencies capable of serving the developmentally disabled adult
2. Knowledge of techniques in using these human resources to enhance the quality of the client's life
3. Acquisition and/or upgrading of teaching skills.
4. Acquisition and/or upgrading of the information on human growth and development as it related to the client
5. Acquisition and/or upgrading of the techniques of a helping relationship

The training program was maximized by inviting guest lecturers for the weekly seminars. These seminar guest speakers were presented in addition to the sessions by the two university professors. Visitations were also arranged to appropriate sites where relevant experiences were shared.

The selection of the client by the advocate was accomplished on a purely affective basis. A social gathering was held at which the two groups interacted freely. On the basis of this meeting, the advocates, and in some instances the prospective clients, indicated the person with whom they preferred to work. The end product of the screening and training process for the prospective advocate was to present to each client a paraprofessional person who was capable of maximizing his or her life chances through effective interaction on both behavioral and affective levels.

Activities with Developmentally Disabled Adults

Advocates taught clients skills and provided them with growth-producing experiences in a large number of activities, including the following.

Teaching Skills for Daily Living

1. Grooming, clothing care, and coordination. This included personal hygiene, use of makeup, hair care, clothing selection, coordination, repair, and care.
2. Traveling skills. This included location of pertinent resource agencies, major shopping areas, bus and taxi transportation skills.

3. Basic communication skills. This area of instruction included appropriate telephone communication behaviors, letter writing, and the use of postal services.
4. Consumer skills. Clients were taught money management (e.g., coin and bill denominations, use of banking, and writing of checks). In addition, shopping skills were emphasized (e.g., reading newspaper ads, observing sales, and coordinating clothing).

But the senoir advocates did far more than simply teach community survival skills to their clients. Recognizing the importance of the affective domain in the overall development of the client and being aware that the developmentally disabled adults had been institutionalized from 2 to 27 years, a major emphasis was placed on social reintegration into the life of the community through the utilization of existing recreation and cultural resources. It was hoped that the developmentally disabled adult, receiving an exposure on several occasions, would remember and return to these resources as needed in the future.

Socialization

1. Recreational and cultural activities. Recreational activities included visits to centers where arts and crafts were made and exhibited, indoor and outdoor swimming activities, attendance at major sports events and dances, and visits to relatives. In addition, parties celebrating major events on the calendar were planned and held by and for the clients (e.g., Halloween, Christmas, Valentine's Day). Cultural activities were also planned and engaged in including attendance at various local theater events (e.g., musicals, ice-skating shows), musical events, and visits to museums and local factories. As part of this socialization process, clients were taken to restaurants, where they were instructed in use of menus, table manners, skills in ordering food, and money management.
2. Altruism. It is regarded as vital that a person learn to give of himself or herself to those less fortunate. Aside from the significance of raising self-esteem for the client, altruism is viewed as one major component of appropriate community relations. Hence, developmentally disabled adult clients were encouraged by the senior advocates to help less fortunate

persons through activities, including the construction of Halloween and Easter baskets for children at a local hospital, the planning of parties for children, and the development of Christmas cards and books for handicapped and/or hospitalized youngsters.

Advocacy

In addition to the above, the older workers engaged in various kinds of advocacy on behalf of the developmentally disabled adult. They reported to the Association for Retarded Citizens regarding responsiveness, concern, and abilities of the various facilities to whom the developmentally disabled adult clients had been released. In addition, they initiated activities which culminated in peridontal and other dental care and improved health care and which provided the developmentally disabled adults with opportunities to practice better personal hygiene (e.g., examinations for lice and ticks). The senior advocates found ways to provide their clients with appropriate and adequate seasonal clothing, encouraged them to learn and practice better nutrition and health habits (e.g., weight control under the supervision of a physician), and advocated and helped the developmentally disabled adults to obtain and manage their own money (including using banking facilities).

Conclusions

The senior advocates all felt that they had made a significant contribution. Although no empirical tests were administered prior to the program, all of the senior advocates reported they felt better physically, had a heightened self-esteem, had increasing self-confidence, and felt sadness that the program was terminating. Some reported they would like to continue with similar activities. Some also mentioned the "good" feelings they experienced when they had to go to college (i.e., workshop and visitation of other ongoing programs). The directors made an emphatic recommendation, based on their observations and work with other adults, that there should be encouragement for the development of similar programs to train older persons for worthwhile paid employment or meaningful volunteering.

References

Boaz, A. *Cost-Benefit Study of the Foster Grandparent Program.* Administrative Services, Washington, D.C., June 1, 1972.

Greenleigh Associates, New York. *An Evaluation of the Foster Grandparent Program.* Office of Economic Opportunity, Washington, D.C., October 1966.

Kalson, L. MASH, a program of social interaction between institutionalized aged and adult mentally retarded person. *The Gerontologist,* 1976, *4*, 340–348.

National Association for Retarded Citizens. By-laws 1974.

Nooe, R. Toward independent living for the mentally retarded. *Social Work,* 1975, *20*, 286–290.

Richards, B. W. Modern perspective in the psychology of old age. In J. G. Howells (ed.), *Mental Retardation in Modern Perspective in the Psychiatry of Old Age.* New York: Brunner, Stash, and Mazel, 1975.

Rosow, I. The social context of the aging self. *The Gerontologist,* 1973, *13*, 82–87.

Rynerson, B. C. Need for self-esteem in the aged: A literature review. *Journal of Psychiatric Nursing and Mental Health Services,* 1972, *10*, 22–26.

Schapiro, J., and Grob, P. *Senior Advocacy Program and the Developmentally Disabled Adult.* Developmental Disabilities Planning and Advisory Council of Virginia, February 1976.

Segal, R. M. *Proceedings: A Consultation-Conference on the Gerontological Aspect of Mental Retardation.* April 8–10, 1975.

5

The Grandparent as an Advocate in Mexican-American Culture

Michael P. Tristan
Ruth M. Bakke

Some cultures within American society define old age as having its onset chronologically earlier in life than age 65. These same cultural groups tend to attribute to the elderly a special status and social usefulness. Black, Mexican-American, and American Indian elderly all have lowered life expectancy rates attributed largely to socioeconomic deprivation (Butler, 1975). There is evidence that blacks generally tend to define old age at an earlier chronological date. This is said to be true of Mexicans and Mexican-Americans as well. Among Mexican-American women, "oldness" is dated from the time the last child marries and leaves the home (Diaz-Guerrero, 1975). Generally, parents whose children are grown and married are considered "*viejitos*"—little old ones. In a society which accepts the brevity of life as a reality, chronological age is of little significance, and in such cultures the elderly are generally held in high esteem. Indeed, the older individuals are sought out as sources of advice and counsel by the young (Clark, 1970; Diaz-Guerrero, 1975).

The sense of *familismo* is a strong component of Mexican-American culture in urban and rural areas (Clark, 1970; Grebler, Moore, and Guzman, 1970; Madsen, 1964; Rubel, 1966). As a part of this commitment, respect and devotion to the elders of the family is an almost constant attribute of the Mexican-American young. Clark cogently describes the group decision making regarding health matters of an individual by the nuclear and extended families (Clark, 1970). Indeed, this at times becomes the augmented family, by virtue of the fact of *compadrazgo* relationships, which constitute functional families among persons who may or may not be kin. The group decisions, thus, are often influenced by the elders in any given extended or augmented family system. A child requiring elective adenoidectomy because of obstructive middle ear disease is likely to undergo such surgery if, and only if, the parents receive the social sanction for granting permission for the operation from sisters, brothers, cousins, *comadres, compadres,* parents, aunts and uncles, and other persons with an interest in the family system.

We had the opportunity to establish and operate a comprehensive health care project for children and youth in a rural south Texas geographic region in which acculturation from traditional Mexican family value systems had not occurred to any great extent. In the process of developing outreach services for the children and youth of these communities, we attempted to tap into the strength of the older citizens, utilizing their knowledge of the family networks in their communities, to assist as advocates and facilitators for the children served by the project. This seemed a natural thing to do, given the cultural factors impinging upon the community, since the children and youth were still a part of the generally accepted cultural value system.

A description of the setting is followed by a discussion of the Children and Youth Program, the development of the project described here, and our attempts to establish the older persons in the geographic area as facilitators and advocates of the health of the young. There was a precedent for this approach, as others have included care and teaching of the younger child as appropriate potential activities for the elderly (Streib, 1971).

Description of the Setting

The Children and Youth Project was established in 1970 in a 200-square-mile rural area in Texas near the center of a semicircular catchment area bounded on the east by the Gulf of Mexico, on the south and southwest by the Rio Grande, and on the northwest and north by an expanse of virtually unpopulated land. The region is characterized by (1) a predominantly Mexican-American population, (2) a striking income variation most adverse for the Mexican-American population, (3) a predominantly agrarian economy, and (4) marked socioeconomic deprivation. The project area varied from this general description only in that the population was, if anything, more disenfranchised. The major population center, a town of some 18,000 population, had originally been the home base for a large number of migrant farm laborers. At the time the project began, much of this population was destitute because of almost total mechanization of the agricultural work formerly performed by hand. Little, if any, industrialization had occurred to offset this lack of employment opportunity.

The population of the target area was 22,000 (90 percent Mexican-American, 8 percent black American, 2 percent all others). Most annual median family incomes were well below poverty levels: the average family size was 7.5 persons and the average annual income was slightly under $2,000. Outside of identified towns, most families lived in small groups and enclaves, either in small entrepreneurial farm communities or in shacks or cabins lining farm-to-market roads and drainage ditches. Isolation of these augmented families was extreme. Many complex social problems existed ranging from the intense isolation and poverty of thinly populated agrarian rural areas with all the attendant lack of social, educational, and health facilities, to the urban "culture of poverty" characterizing the major population centers of south Texas and the Texas/Mexico border. Throughout the region, binguality and variance from traditional white Caucasian-American values added burdens which made the delivery of adequate social and health services a task of seemingly insurmountable difficulty.

Medical care prior to the project was provided by eight private general practitioners, three of whom were at or beyond retirement age. Dental services were virtually nonexistent. A county hospital district and a charity children's hospital were located from 25 to 75 miles from families served by the project. The eligibility guidelines of these two institutions ensured the exclusion of many residents of the target area who qualified as "working poor."

Medical problems encountered were those expected—acute and chronic infectious diseases, malnutrition, failure to thrive, and developmental and psychosocial problems among the children. Hospitalization of children and youth of the target area for some or all of these conditions was the rule. In addition, there had been considerable inpatient experience with neonatal problems, due largely to the lack of relevant obstetrical services, with the consequent dependence on indigenous services.

Background of the Children and Youth Program and Children and Youth Project 660

Title V of the Social Security Act of 1935 provided for grants to the states for maternal and child welfare administered through the Children's Bureau. In 1963, Public Law 88–156 included amendments to Title V authorizing special project grants for comprehensive maternal and infant care and in 1965 Public Law 89-97 authorized additional special project grants for the children and youth (C&Y) programs (Wilson and Neuhauser, 1974). The establishment of these complimentary programs was the culmination of thirty years of planning by the Children's Bureau aimed at providing comprehensive and continuous care to low-income families from the prenatal period to young adulthood (Lesser, 1970). It was generally acknowledged that many preschool and school age children and youth of low-income families did not receive adequate medical attention (U.S. House, 1965).

The special children and youth projects were designed to

provide comprehensive health services for children in low income families through promotion of health as well as medical care, including case finding, preventive health services, diagnosis, treatment, correction of defects and after care, both medical and dental. The emphasis is to be placed on the comprehensiveness and continuity of services (DHEW, 1965).

Continuity of care was to be insured by the progress of clients through a health care process starting with registration, proceeding through an assessment of care needs and the rendering of necessary services, to the maintenance of an "optimal" level of health for the individual. Comprehensiveness was to be obtained by having registrants assessed and given care when needed by nine disciplines: medicine, dentistry, nursing, nutrition, social work, psychology, speech and hearing, physical therapy, and occupational therapy. New methods of providing care to children were to be developed, tested, and applied (Green, 1969). In this sense, the individual children and youth projects were intended to be "demonstrations" (Ouradnik and Weckworth, 1970).

The planning and initiation of the detailed proposal for the south Texas project was begun in the summer and early fall of 1969. Funding began on May 1, 1970, with a teaching hospital as the grantee agency.

Major efforts initially were directed toward recruiting core staff, refining operational plans, developing in-service educational programs, and organizing the physical plant for the facility in the target area. However, care for identified patients from the target area was begun (as staff were recruited) even before renovation of the physical plant in the target area was completed. Location and preparation of the facility was complete by January 1971. All children and youth from birth through 16 years of age residing within the geographic area defined were eligible for screening, diagnosis, and preventive services. Treatment, correction of defects, and aftercare were available to children who met the specific means tests of the grantee hospital with exceptions made under special circumstances of medical or social need. In these instances, the project director approved such patients for project care after due consultation with core staff, the health care teams of the clinical facility, and appropriate consultants. A core staff group was established which included the chief of each of the disciplines involved, the project director, and the project administrator. Major policy decisions regarding project operations were arrived at largely by consensus of this group. In three years only two major policy decisions had to be made directly by the project director because of lack of consensus within the core staff. One of those policy decisions was the decision to establish a consumer council.

Development of the Consumer Council

Unlike the early Office of Economic Opportunity neighborhood health centers, the individual C&Y projects were not required by statute or regulations to develop a governing council which would include consumers (DHEW, 1965). Most projects were encouraged by DHEW to develop such councils for feedback of information from the target population. From its earliest days, C&Y Project 660 envisioned such a consumer council. As core staff were recruited and operations began, the issue of establishing a consumer council was raised at core staff meetings. The debate intensified and became more acrimonious as time went by, lasting more than a year before the project director took definitive action. No consensus was ever reached. Interestingly, members of the core staff all polarized early, either for or against such a council. Representatives from nursing, social work, psychology, nutrition, and education supported the concept. Those against the formation of such a council were administration, medicine, dentistry, and physical medicine and rehabilitation. Those opposed to the idea were the most adamant and vociferous in their arguments. Their concern seems to have been that the consumer council would in some way gain decision-making control of the project. The individual core staff members were not reassured by the project director's continuing insistence that he did not intend to delegate authority for project operations to such a consumer council. Indeed, such delegation would have been contrary to regulations. Supporters had worked out a number of highly structured activities for such a council, in addition to serving as sources of information relative to project operations. The major of these was to develop the system of neighborhood aides or child advocates which is the subject of this report. Additionally, functions included supervision of an adolescent program which would include volunteers within the clinic, development of a supervised play area for siblings of children attending the clinic, assistance with redecorating clinic rooms and examination areas, and a program to motivate adolescents and young adults in the community to pursue careers in health services.

The project director decided by fiat in late 1972 that a consumer council would be established. The leadership role in the development of such a council was carried by the nursing and social work staffs following the structured lines discussed in the many debates among the core staff. Throughout the early months of 1973, there was an intensive effort to screen parents, grandparents, and relatives of patients of the clinic for persons considered to be reasonable and effective community participants and to identify those willing and able to actively serve on such a consumer council. By mid-May, a group of 13 persons, all women, had been identified and regular meetings established. The neighborhood aide/child advocate project was the initial and most important project undertaken by the council and began almost immediately after the organizing meetings.

The most important topic discussed by the consumers themselves was the militancy of certain radical political groups in the community: they denounced these groups and assured project staff of their devotion and commitment to the project and its activities in the target area. It is interesting to note that militancy had been considered as one reason for not establishing a consumer council. It had been repeatedly pointed out that the severe poverty of the target area was such that little energy was available on the part of most of the consumers for any significant level of militant social activity. Input from social work and nursing was intense and required a great deal of effort to overcome the council members' initial reluctance to voice any criticism of project services.

Once a relatively homogeneous working group of parents, grand-parents, and others had been established, the council proceeded to establish its neighborhood aide/child advocacy program. The goals of the program were to provide outreach to unserved potential registrants, improve the scope and quality as well as the continuity of care received by current registrants, and reorient parents/consumers away from acute crisis episodic care to health supervision and preventive services. Of significance is that the older workers involved had a great deal to do with the success of the program.

The Older Worker in the Advocacy Role

Of the women identified as "concerned parents" with an interest in the concept of a consumer council, 5 were young (25 or under, including one unwed adolescent mother), 5 were aged 26–40, and the remainder were over 41 years of age. Of those who remained on the council, the majority (60 percent) were classified as "older workers," i.e., in their community they were considered to be elders, valued for their wisdom. They had attained such status by virtue of influence on their extended and augmented families. Four of these will be used as examples.

Ms. P., aged 64, was a great-grandparent, having raised several children of her own and several grandchildren due to the untimely death of her son. She continued to be active in the nurturing of her great-grandchildren even at some distance. None of her grandchildren were project registrants but she had been the unofficial foster parent for innumerable children over the years, and many of these children were cared for by the project. She was the only black member of the council and became a very vocal and outspoken representative of the small but closely knit black community within the target area. Ms. P. was the true neighborhood matriarch. She was consulted by the younger generation for all manners of social, spiritual, and health problems. She had for some years served as an unofficial day care center, offering succorance to her many charges far surpassing the accepted role of "baby-sitter." Her methods were generally viewed by the project staff to be very unorthodox but highly effective.

Ms. P. was able to actively serve black project registrants since the black population of the target area was sequestered in a fairly small area and virtually all of the families were known to her. In addition, she was an active participant in the church attended by most of the black participants, and she worked closely with a variety of church groups as well as other civic groups with black representation. She was extremely supportive and positive about the Children and Youth Project and its accomplishments and remained active and faithful to the project in community circles.

Ms. S. P. was in her mid-40s and was a Mexican-American mother of children ranging in ages from their early 20s to the youngest at age 3 who suffered from residual brain damage as a result of viral encephalitis. She was the best educated of the council members, having attained the status of a licensed vocational nurse. She was not working at the time of her involvement with the council because of the time and effort required for her handicapped child. She and her family were well known in the community and were active in many activities. Because of her status as an LVN and her experience with her handicapped child, she was often consulted by younger parents regarding problems of their own.

Ms. S. C., a Mexican-American woman in her late 40s, was the one individual who almost single-handedly held the consumer council together. She had a great interest in the project and was quick to support and suggest any activities that might enhance its effectiveness. She had many children of her own who were well known to the clinic staff and a husband who was very willing to offer assistance with any projects requiring manual labor. Because of her activities in her local church group, she was able to enlist the aid and assistance of many other persons and families who did not have children eligible for care in the performance of planned activities. The unexpected result was that community involvement from many sources outside the immediate families cared for by the project was initiated.

Ms. R., a 72-year-old Mexican-American inactive indigenous midwife, came to the attention of project staff through her involvement with a number of children to whom she was related by blood or compadrazgo ties. Her own children were all grown, so that project-identified blood relatives were grandchildren and great-grandchildren. Ms. R. had ceased functioning as a local midwife some 10–15 years prior to the establishment of the project because of "lots of trouble with the authorities [Public Health Department Prenatal and Perinatal Service personnel] over such things as medicines for the mothers and sickness among the babies." She indicated that continuing to practice her profession after 40 years "was not worth it." Furthermore, while she had learned her profession from an elder *partera* in the small south Texas community where she grew up, she noted that none of the young women of the current generation were interested in following in her footsteps. "They all want to go to college to be nurses," she would say, sadly, bitterly. Because she was well known and highly respected in the community, her participation in the advocacy program was considered to be highly desirable. She functioned in a marginal way, however, being somewhat limited by her cynicism about the project and its staff. She was able, however, to identify elder women in many geographic subareas who subsequently participated.

Around this nucleus the social work and nursing staffs developed the advocacy program. Members of the council were assigned specific geographic areas within the largest population center and in the remainder of the rural target area. An attempt was made to tailor these geographic areas to the known social networks of the council members. The council itself was called on to recruit others in positions of influence in geographic areas without council representation. The activities of the council members serving in the advocacy role were then defined and prioritized as (1) follow-up of missed appointments, (2) setting of appointments for children not previously registered for health assessment and preventive services, and (3) identification of others within the community able to assist in the advocacy facilitator role.

Inherent in the role of the advocate was conveying to project staff the attitudes of parents and children served by the clinic regarding those services. Additionally, their activity led to the identification of a number of rather major mental health problems that had not been identified previously. In this area, advocate facilitators' primary contact personnel were social work case aides integral to the project's health care teams. They also attempted to develop community activities through other community agencies such as the PTA, schools, and churches. Not all of these activities were initially seen as high priority, but they tended to occur spontaneously.

In the spring of 1973, the neighborhood aides and child advocates entered a familiarization and training program developed jointly by the nursing and social work staffs. By early summer, the group began to be active in the field. Throughout the summer of 1973 staff reported a positive effect in terms of follow-up on missed appointments and a small but definite increase in project growth rate was recorded (4.55 percent in April, May, June to 5.29 percent in July, August, and September). Simultaneously, major administrative changes began to take place in the grantee agency which seriously affected the functioning of the project. By the fall of 1973, a series of administrative changes were made which resulted in an almost complete changeover in the project core staff from those who had been present at the time the project was funded. The result was that the social work and nursing staff increasingly limited their involvement with the council members and with the advocacy group, and when key project core staff members left, all advocate facilitator activities ceased. It was never entirely clear as to what extent these older workers acted as child advocates and to what extent their role was facilitative.

Discussion

It is clear that the foregoing comments regarding the older worker as a child advocate are anecdotal. A data system which might have provided some information regarding the effect of the child advocate program on project operations was in place but terminated within a year of the establishment of the program. In addition, the administrative difficulties previously described occurred within three months of the establishment of the child advocacy program and additional data thereafter were not forthcoming.

The perceived goals of the child advocacy program included the following:

1. Develop outreach to children and youth not presently served by the project
2. Establish appropriate continuity of care including the provision of acute, chronic, health supervision, and routine preventive services
3. Establish a change in utilization patterns from acute crisis-oriented care to comprehensive care with emphasis on provision of routine preventive services, parenting skills, and health education
4. Establish communication linkages between the project and existing curing and caring health networks within the community (midwives and faith healers, as well as existing institutions and agencies), and
5. Expand health education activities

Available data clearly indicate that the project provided a source of significant services to the children and youth of the target area (Tristan, 1975). Staff observations and a small but definite increase in the project's growth rate suggest that the child advocacy program contributed to the total services provided.

It was felt that the role of the older worker as a child advocate was socially and culturally congruent. The interest generated within the community in serving on the Consumer Council and with the project as a child advocate was exclusively on the part of the women. The older woman is performing "women's work" when she looks after the health and welfare of the young. Additionally, the older women in Mexican and Mexican-American communities are known to wield considerable influence in their families, neighborhoods, and communities. Finally, there were practical reasons for attempting to recruit older workers. Most older workers in the geographic area were unemployable because of the relatively high unemployment rates among the younger population and because of their general lack of marketable skills. Thus, a fairly large pool of available labor was present and required only recruitment and training.

In summary, anecdotal experience suggests that the advocacy system utilizing older workers was effective. Indeed, the advocacy/facilitator program seemed to those of us involved more as a recognition, institutionalization, and formalization of an existing cultural state of affairs. Had the program survived, we believe that it would not only have provided an increase of the scope of high-quality services to a significant population of children and youth but would also have represented a positive outreach to the elderly of the community.

References

Butler, R. N. *Why Survive? Being Old in America*. New York: Harper and Row, 1975.

Clark, M. *Health in the Mexican American Culture*. Berkeley: University of California Press, 1970.

Diaz-Guerrero, R. *Psychology of the Mexican*. Austin: University of Texas Press, 1975.

Grebler, L., Moore, J. W., and Guzman, R. C. *The Mexican American People*. New York: Free Press, 1970.

Green, G. *Calculating the Cost of Delivering Comprehensive Health Care in*

Children and Youth Projects: A Conceptual Model and a Case Study.
Systems Development Project Comment Series, N 9–10, 1969.

Lesser, A. D. Presentation to the meeting of dental directors of children and youth projects, Detroit, Michigan, May 2, 1970.

Madsen, W. *The Mexican Americans of South Texas.* San Francisco: Holt, Rinehart and Winston, 1964.

Ouradnik, N., and Weckworth, V. E. *Some Unique Aspects of the Children and Youth Projects.* Systems Development Project Comment Series, N 0–8, 1970.

Rubel, A. J. *Across the Tracks: Mexican Americans in a Texas City.* Austin: University of Texas Press, 1966.

Streib, G. F. New roles and activities for retirement. In G. L. Maddox (ed.), *The Future of Aging and the Aged.* Atlanta: Southern Newspaper Publishers Association Foundation, 1971.

Tristan, M. P. *Pitfalls in Health Services Research in the Operational Setting: A Study of the Effect of a Comprehensive Ambulatory Clinical Facility in a Rural Area on the Utilization of In-Hospital Services.* Unpublished thesis, University of Texas School of Public Health, 1975.

U.S. Department of Health, Education and Welfare: Children's Bureau, Grants for Comprehensive Health Services for Children and Youth, Policies and Procedures, 1965.

U.S. House of Representatives, Committee on Ways and Means, Social Security Amendments of 1965, Report of the Committee on Ways and Means on House Report 6673, House #213, 89th Congress, 1st Session.

Wilson, F. A., and Neuhauser, D. *Health Services in the United States.* Cambridge, Mass.: Ballinger, 1974.

Part III

Benefits and Limitations of the Use of Older Workers/Volunteers

6

The Older (Indigenous) Worker: Assets and Problems

Rosemary McCaslin
Nancy Wilson

The Rise of Paraprofessionalism

During the past two decades there has been widespread interest among both theoreticians and practitioners in the helping professions in the feasibility of utilizing paraprofessional personnel to extend the availability and reduce the cost of services (e.g., Austin, 1977; Barg and Hirsch, 1972; Barker and Briggs, 1968; Epstein, 1962; Gershon and Biller, 1977; Heyman, 1966; Richan, 1961; Weed and Denham, 1961). In the United States this trend appears to have been augmented by the convergence of several economic, social, and educational developments.

1. Spiraling inflation has rapidly increased the cost of professional services with no accompanying increase in the availability of funds for their support. In fact, social services have often been among the first curtailed in attempts to control government spending.
2. At the same time, there has been increased awareness of the necessity to provide supports throughout the life span for persons living in complex postindustrial societies. More and more services have come to be accepted as essential "social

An earlier version of this chapter appeared in the Administration on Aging's magazine, *Aging,* May–June 1980 (Nos. 307–308), pp. 24–29.

utilities" (Kahn, 1969) and the roles deemed appropriate to
government have expanded accordingly. This has been especially true in relation to the needs of older persons as that group
has become a larger proportion of the total population[1] and has
concomitantly become more visible and vocal.

3. The combination of these countervailing forces has created
   strong pressures on service providers to account for their use of
   public funds in terms of both the effectiveness and efficiency of
   their programs. Traditional practice models have often been
   found less than satisfactory regarding both cost/benefit criteria
   and the degree of community control they allow.

4. The War on Poverty of the 1960s attempted to draw more
   heavily on the capacity of communities to generate their own
   solutions to social and economic problems and called attention
   to the value of experiential understanding of subcultural
   phenomena. The ultimate success of that movement has been
   rather limited, but its failure stemmed more from inadequate
   funding and contradictory political objectives than from problems with its theoretical base (e.g., Greenstone and Peterson,
   1973). An enduring contribution from that period has been
   recognition of the indigenous paraprofessional as a vital link in
   human service delivery and an increased awareness of the need
   to reevaluate the role of the professional social worker vis-a-vis
   the goal of mobilizing the client's capacity for corrective action
   in his or her own behalf.

5. Educators have responded to these pressures by giving increased emphasis to specification of basic practitioner competencies
   and development of briefer curricula capable of attaining those
   objectives (e.g., Baer and Federico, 1978; CSWE, 1976a and b).
   Not only has the necessity of graduate education been questioned in some professions, but subbaccalaureate training
   programs have been increasingly considered as options.

To date, most examinations of the special contributions of indigenous paraprofessionals have focused on workers slected from poverty
and/or minority groups. Yet, if the concept is valid, i.e., if experiential
understanding of special problem areas is as important as theoretical
understanding, then the indigenous qualities of many other groups of
persons should be of value in the provision of human services. In
practice this has long been recognized, e.g., commissions for the blind
hire many blind persons, rehabilitation programs hire handicapped

persons. To some extent programs for the elderly have also tended to utilize the talents of the people they serve, but this too often has been seen as "allowing" the aged to participate or "giving" them something to do. And in some instances the economic objectives of liberating low-income older persons from poverty have been emphasized to the extent that the worker's skills are completely discounted. There has been almost no consideration of the unique contributions which older workers can make to programs for the elderly based on their being "indigenous," i.e., possessing an experiential understanding of problems common in old age.

It has been the experience of these authors that the use of older paraprofessionals as geriatric mental health workers not only is economically advantageous but also can enhance the effectiveness of the total program of which they are a part. This chapter outlines the assets and problems which a group of older workers have added to the process of service delivery as a result of their indigenous character-istics—being of the same age and/or life stage, race, class, sex, and community identification as the clients they are attempting to help.

A Programmatic Example

Texas Research Institute of Mental Sciences (TRIMS), located in the Texas Medical Center in Houston, is the research and training facility of the Texas Department of Mental Health and Mental Retardation. The institute also functions as a direct-service provider in order to maintain contact with clinical populations necessary to its research and training roles and to develop and evaluate treatment/service delivery models as one of its research contributions. The geriatric section of the institute has been developed over the past 10 years to include a comprehensive mental health program ranging from preventive com-munity services to inpatient and outpatient treatment of emotional and/ or psychiatric disorders, backed up by biological, medical, and psycho-social research capacities. Program staff play important leadership roles in the development of health and social services for older persons throughout the community and the state.

TRIMS' geriatric program has always stressed the capacity of the majority of elderly clients to make their own problem-solving decisions when allowed to do so and given adequate information and support. Considerable effort has been directed at reversing the tendency of both laypersons and professionals to infantilize the elderly by doing everything for them. When an opportunity arose to create part-time paraprofessional positions within the service, staff felt they had a responsibility to "practice what they preached" and to seek out older persons to fill those positions.

In January 1974, 4 older women were hired to extend existing information and referral services to community-based nutrition/activity sites for the elderly to whom TRIMS had a service responsibility. Based on positive experience in that initial program, 5 additional older women were subsequently hired as field workers for an aftercare/alternate care service begun July 1974. Evaluation of the contributions of these first 9 older workers led to the conclusion that the model warranted expansion, and 2 additional paraprofessional positions were created in April 1976. Currently, the Senior Information and Outreach Program of TRIMS has all of its 11 part-time positions filled by older workers. Two of these are women in their late 40s, 2 men and 3 women are in their late 50s, 2 women are in their 60s, and 2 women are in their 70s.[2]

All paraprofessional staff initially receive about a month of intensive orientation to agency functions and procedures, community resources, and normal and abnormal aging processes. Throughout their employment, they are involved in in-service training through weekly staff meetings and opportunities to attend various special meetings and conferences. Their immediate supervisors, who are experienced B.A. and M.A. level social workers, meet with the workers in regular individual sessions to discuss active cases and specific problems encountered in the field. These supervisors carry primary responsibility for the workers, but all other members of the multidisciplinary staff are called on as appropriate for training and consultation. Additionally, paraprofessionals work directly with the psychiatrists, social workers, psychologists, and nurses on the clinical staff with whom they share responsibility for specific cases and benefit from their insights both in private discussions and in case conferences.

Older workers provide information and resource counseling to elderly residents of assigned neighborhoods throughout the county, establishing community bases in existing loci such as congregate dining sites, health clinics, and nursing homes. They not only make themselves readily accessible to older persons at these places but also play a case-finding role, interacting within the ongoing flow of center or clinic activity with an eye open for yet unstated problems. They work closely with supervisory staff to assess whether to provide clients with direct supportive services or to focus their efforts on enabling the client to use TRIMS' clinical facilities. Additionally, they are used as extensors of professional services, making home visits to monitor health status progress and providing continuity between clinic visits and/or following hospitalization. The older workers' functions, then, are geared toward integrating and increasing the accessibility of all other agency services, making the total program different than it would be without their input.

Evaluating the Older Worker's Contribution

The costs and benefits involved in using older workers in a geriatric mental health program such as TRIMS' are difficult to separate clearly. The very qualities that enable an older person to make unique and important contributions to the agency's efforts are often the source of new problems for supervisory personnel. One must consider the addition of older paraprofessionals to an agency staff as a qualitative change in programming, creating a new set of supervisory tasks along with a new set of service potentialities.

Orientation to the Helping Role

Few of the older workers hired at TRIMS had had any human service experience in a professional agency setting or previous experience in working with the elderly. However, the past experiences of the workers had afforded them considerable contact with individuals and their communities. The vocational backgrounds represented among these staff included teaching, journalism, barbering, and military service, and several workers had been active as volunteers and participants in community affairs. The primary criteria for their selection were their ability to relate well to other people, their positive attitudes toward aging, and their own interest in community work with older persons.[3]

As anticipated, the older workers show a special ability to understand and relate to the problems of elderly clients. Their own age and experience with life in the respective communities of their clients seem to contribute to their abilities to understand and develop effective helping relationships. The close identification of these workers with their clients often leads to a tendency to pursue solutions with a vigor, urgency, and persistence not as commonly found among their younger colleagues. It is almost as if they are driven at times by a feeling of "there but for the grace of God go I." This greater investment in client outcomes among the older workers often leads to more extensive collaboration among different levels of staff than had existed previously.

Not having an extensive theoretical base from which to work, however, their frame of reference is primarily their own experience and that of persons they have known. Attempts at generalized conceptual learning in supervision and in-service training are often met with an insistence on focusing on the familiar particular and avoiding consideration of alternative possibilities. Each worker will try to center the discussion on his or her "favorite" client (usually the person in his or her current caseload with whom he or she is most able to identify) and resist attempts to explore the similarities in human dynamics among the externally different clients. The danger of overidentification with client problems and failure to adequately individualize each situation is ever present.

It has also been noted that because older workers are keenly aware of the impact of negative American cultural attitudes and social and economic practices on the lives of older people, they often focus on the external realities of a client's problems without identifying internal difficulties or intrapsychic problems. Supervision and training which emphasize the psychological aspects of given case situations are necessary to sensitize the older worker to these levels of problem analysis.

The older worker's difficulty in maintaining some objective distance from a given client's situation may result in certain options for intervention being overlooked and/or an overwhelming amount of frustration to be managed by the worker when ready solutions for the problems are not apparent. This problem is certainly not unique to older paraprofessionals, but does seem to be exacerbated by the need many of them feel to validate the accumulated experiences of a lifetime. This is somewhat offset (happily breaking stereotypes) by an eagerness to take advantage of opportunities for gaining completely new knowledge and skills late in life.

Age and Community Identification

The older workers bring an advantage with age in feeling a greater freedom to confront clients regarding their behavior. It is much more difficult for elderly clients, for example, to justify withdrawal from activity because of age when the workers confronting them are as old or older than the clients. The factor of community identification enters the picture: the workers' freedom based on age role to confront clients is increased by the sanction that comes from working in the community of which they are a part and in which they have the sanction of personal status. Older people in particular are learned historians of their own community and its members. An older worker's knowledge of significant landmarks and his or her own personal status as a fellow resident may be the critical factors in the establishment of good worker/client rapport. On the other hand, an older worker who has been a community activist may be hampered in helping effectiveness by a need to defend against loss of personal status, should a given client reject the worker's viewpoint. It has become necessary to take into account the subgroup identification of the individual worker within the grass roots structure of the community when making field assignments because of the effect of such personal identifications on the worker's potential effectiveness.

The visibility of older persons among the staff has made the service less threatening and more readily acceptable to many potential clients. The older workers are able to explain the services of the agency and their statements are accepted as "trustworthy" by elderly persons who are unfamiliar with and suspicious of mental health services. This same phenomenon seems to operate with some agencies which have initially misunderstood or distrusted TRIMS' motives. Grass roots organizations and agencies staffed largely by paraprofessionals seem to trust the statements of older mental health workers, who display concern for their older client's needs as well as the problems of the overall community. More established community agencies and those staffed primarily by professionals, however, sometimes react skeptically to the older workers. The skepticism seems to arise from the ongoing struggle between professionals and paraprofessionals and some ageism on the part of those individuals who view older people as unable to perform as effective mental health workers.

At a quite different level, a supervisory task has emerged which seems unique to working with older paraprofessionals. To one extent or another, most of these workers have been affected by the lowered self-esteem so often imposed on the aging person in this society. Furthermore, the older workers may face some of the same social and physiological problems which they encounter among their clients, such as loss of significant others, decline in physical health. In order for the older worker to maintain the confidence necessary to master new knowledge, learn new roles, and continue to perform his or her tasks effectively, these personal problems must be understood and dealt with. Supervision must in some instances include therapeutic elements and assistance with personal problems encountered by the aging worker. Yet it has been found that, often, more is accomplished "therapeutically" by keeping such therapeutics to a minimum. Reasonable expectations for transcendence and continued job performance seem to be of greatest benefit in enhancing the older worker's ability to solve problems.

Equally as important as the older workers' ability to deal with elderly clients have been the benefits the mental health team has derived from their addition to the staff. The presence of older workers and their unique perspective on aging provides a constant self-correcting influence for younger professionals on the team. The older workers are equally quick to point out occasions when the perspectives of other staff members do or do not agree with their own experiences.

Staff become less likely to make sweeping and invalid generalizations and often obtain invaluable in-service information unavailable through other sources, such as insight into adjusting to dentures. Just as the clients benefit from the positive role model of these active older workers, so do other staff members benefit from their daily exposure to successful aging.

Ethnicity and Sex Roles

The close community and ethnic ties of the older workers described here must also be recognized as major factors affecting their job performance: age is not the only characteristic relevant to worker/client identification.

Both the paraprofessionals and their professional coworkers on TRIMS' staff are triethnic (Anglo, black, and Mexican-American) corresponding to the population of the community. For many of the older workers, this is their first experience in working closely with persons from differing cultural perspectives. Acting as advocates for the unique qualities of their own group, they force all staff members to consider important factors that are too easily ignored. Professional staff have been able to gain valuable insights into the needs and perspectives of subgroups of elderly persons through their exposure to the older workers.

Danger of overidentification also grows out of the fact that most of these older workers strongly feel their community and ethnic ties. There is a tendency, for example, for elderly black workers to expect all elderly black clients to view the situation as they do. And when this does not occur, an overly identifying worker may develop punitive or rejecting behavior toward the client. This problem has been more easily dealt with as the triethnic paraprofessional staff size increases and there are more opportunities to exchange personal accounts about what it is like, for example, to be black.

It should be noted that the same cultural ties that are assets in other instances at times present barriers to the worker's effectiveness. Certain cultural norms are too strong to be abridged by the paraprofessional and can substantially affect the courses of action that are open to him or her. For example, it has been impossible for one of our Mexican-American workers to deal with behaviors stemming from sexual identity problems in some of her male clients. In such cases, no amount of supervision has been able to break the barriers imposed on the worker by her own culturally defined roles.

Sex role identification has emerged as deserving attention similar to that afforded ethnic ties. The viewpoints and experiential understanding expressed by two older male workers have been particularly valuable to a predominantly female staff. They have assisted the entire staff in accepting and appreciating the various needs and feelings of an older male toward the aging experience and prevented oversimplified assessments of male clients, such as "He simply misses his work." Furthermore, one of the male workers mobilized significant support from the church denomination of which he was a well-respected leader and the other male worker has educated all staff members in the workings of the Veterans Administration, with which he has negotiated throughout his lifetime. Female workers provide equally valuable personal descriptions of experiences such as familial role reversal from the point of view of a mother. And they, of course, often belong to women's organizations, such as church sisterhoods, which are too easily overlooked by professionals as community resources.

Conclusions

Experience has convinced the authors that older persons can bring to the geriatric mental health team unique and valuable contributions. Their assets stem both from the fact that they themselves are experiencing old age and from the cultural context of their aging.

Lacking formal training in the helping process, older paraprofessionals fall back on the life experiences they have in common with clients and, in so doing, increase the unique contributions they have to offer as indigenous workers. Their more personal approach to client problems creates a set of tasks for their supervisors that are different from those encountered when working with formally trained staff. These are seen, however, as different rather than as additional tasks and are felt to be reasonable efforts to expend in order to effectively use the special attributes of older workers.

In summary, the addition of older persons to the geriatric mental health team has enabled it to reach elderly clients more effectively, has enhanced staff's understanding of different experiences of aging, and has assisted the older persons employed in working through their personal problems. No less important, it has provided a unique means of educating the community and other professionals regarding the potential for continued productivity and fulfillment throughout life. The actions of older persons on the staff speak louder than all good professional words put together.

Notes

1. The proportion of the U.S. population aged 65 and over has increased from 4.1 percent in 1900 to 8.1 percent in 1950 and 10.5 percent in 1975 (Bureau of Census, 1976).

2. Although the program defines older clients as those aged 60 and over, paraprofessional workers are seen as "older" if they are in their late 40s or beyond. Age-based job discrimination is known to begin in mid-life (e.g., the Age Discrimination in Employment Act of 1967 covers workers aged 45–65). Especially for persons lacking special training and skills, the experience of being treated as too old to contribute may begin long before the common retirement age of 65. Because of this, paraprofessional workers in their late 40s or 50s may face problems usually associated with later ages. Additionally, many of the workers discussed here are members of minority communities in which the cultural status of "elder" begins at an earlier age than in the dominant American society. In other ways, of course, these "younger-older workers" are quite different from those in their 60s and 70s.

3. Truax and Carkhuff (1967) established the importance of personality attributes such as empathy, warmth, and genuineness in effective counseling. Such characteristics may be innate or can be produced through training.

References

Austin, M. J. *Professionals and Paraprofessionals.* New York: Human Sciences Press, 1977.

Baer, B. L., and Federico, R. *Educating the Baccalaureate Social Worker: Report of the Undergraduate Social Work Curriculum Project.* Cambridge, Mass.: Ballinger, 1978.

Barg, S. K., and Hirsch, C. A successor model for community support of low-income minority group aged. *Aging and Human Development,* 1972, *3,* 243–252.

Barker, R. L., and Briggs, T. L. *Differential Use of Social Work Manpower.* New York: National Association of Social Workers, 1968.

Bureau of the Census, U.S. Department of Commerce. *Demographic Aspects of Aging and the Older Population in the United States.* Special Studies Series P-23, No. 59, May 1976.

Council on Social Work Education. *Competency-Based Education for Social Work: Evaluation and Curriculum Issues.* New York: CSWE, 1976(a).

Council on Social Work Education. *Teaching for Competence in the Delivery of Direct Services.* New York: CSWE, 1976(b).

Epstein, L. Differential use of staff: A method to expand social services. *Social Work,* 1962, *7,* 66–72.

Gershon, M., and Biller, H. B. *The Other Helpers: Paraprofessionals and Nonprofessionals in Mental Health.* Lexington: Lexington Books, 1977.

Greenstone, J. D., and Peterson, P. E. *Race and Authority in Urban Politics: Community Participation and the War on Poverty.* Chicago: University of Chicago Press, 1973.

Heyman, M. M. Criteria for the allocation of cases according to levels of staff skill. *Social Casework,* 1966, *47,* 325–331.

Kahn, A. J. *Theory and Practice of Social Planning.* New York: Russell Sage Foundation, 1969.

Richan, W. C. A theoretical scheme for determining roles of professional and nonprofessional personnel. *Social Work,* 1961, *6,* 22–28.

Truax, C. G., and Carkhuff, R. R. *Towards Effective Counseling and Psychotherapy.* Chicago: Aldine, 1967.

Weed, V., and Denham, W. H. Toward more effective use of the nonprofessional worker: A recent experiment. *Social Work,* 1961, *6,* 29–36.

7

Denying the Years

Joan Walsh Trelease

Description of Project

During the academic year of 1975–1976 the Program in Gerontology at the University of Rhode Island organized a training program for older people, the Older Advocate Counselors for the Elderly.[1] The objectives of the project were (1) to train well-functioning older adults as advocate counselors for those elderly requiring assistance, (2) to utilize the skills attainable through the project program, (3) to assist the older segment of the community in maintaining independence, and (4) to act as liaisons between the needs of the elderly and the agency best qualified to meet those needs.

The project covered the northern and southern sections of Rhode Island and spanned 12 week periods in the fall and spring. It included 6 weeks of teaching (theory) and 6 weeks of practicum (field experience). To be accepted into the program as a trainee, an applicant had to be 55 years of age or older and have the ability to relate to others regardless of their own standard or ideal of life-style. Those selected for training as older advocates were of varied backgounds. Some were still in the work force but the majority were retired or unemployed. Approximately 80 percent were women: the total sample of finally selected trainees were 25 persons, 5 males and 20 females.

In the teaching phase, meetings were held twice a week. It was found that this approach facilitated understanding by those in the

Funded under the Continuing Education and Community Service Program under Title I of the Higher Education Act of 1965.

program and allowed time for group discussion, study, and role playing. Throughout this period emphasis was placed on (1) assessment and evaluation of age-related problems, (2) availability and utilization of community agencies, and (3) human relations. Five areas in which age-related problems occur were stressed: physical health, emotional health, cognitive abilities, family relations, and present life and the future.

The second or practicum phase involved weekly one-to-one supervision between the trainee and a member of the project staff. These meetings helped resolve areas of concern for the trainees as they became active in some type of community work with the aged.

The Presenting Problem

During the training project the author became aware of an interesting phenomenon—some of the individuals being trained seemed to be denying their true age. Some were open and candid about this fact, others communicated their denial in less obvious ways, e.g., their style of dress, their activities, their associates, and their thinking in reference to their peers.

It is the purpose of this chapter to examine three cases in terms of the meaning of this denial for the individual and the ways in which they used the training program to facilitate their chosen solutions to the role problems reflected in their age denial.

Case Studies

The following case descriptions are of three trainees, each of whom was practicing some form of age denial.

Case 1

Ms. E., a 59-year-old woman for a short period unemployed, had recently regained her position. Her job required work with older people. Ms. E.'s motivation to participate in the project was not only her desire to gain a higher level of skill in working with the elderly but also to maintain her employment. Although she had studied age-related material on her own, she felt she would gain helpful insight through the project study.

When her children no longer needed her at home on a full-time basis, Ms. E. persuaded her husband to agree to her seeking outside employment. It was at this time that she began to deny her age, explaining that "it made it easier for me to find employment." This had seemed a sound and practical reason at the time. Yet now, years later in the training sessions, Ms. E. would refer to people in the target population as those "poor old people," verbally disassociating herself from the aging. The attitudes expressed in her "poor old people" statements reflected an age denial of a personal and deep-rooted nature.

Case 2

Mr. B. was a 60-year-old male who had retired two years previously from Civil Service. Though retired, Mr. B. continued his active role in the union and felt that the experience he had gained from his involvement in union affairs would be very beneficial to him in working with the elderly. His desire to work with the elderly stemmed from his contacts with older people while employed. He felt his participation in the project would allow him to sharpen his skills and facilitate his role as a helper in volunteer activities.

Mr. B. was happy when he retired because he was able to devote his time to achieving his special goal, finishing college. However, when asked if he were retired he admitted that he was, but always added that one could retire at 55 from his field of employment. Although Mr. B. had reaped some benefits from the status as senior citizen, he did not like to be thought of as old. His style of dress reflected a man attempting to recapture youth through "mod" fashion.

Case 3

Ms. R. was a 68-year-old woman who was thought to be 10 years younger by most people in her community. Until a year prior to the project, she had been employed full time as a coordinator of services in a public health agency. She had worked continuously throughout her adult life and her income had contributed to the support of her large family. In recent years, she had remained employed primarily to keep herself active. Having worked in a public health agency, Ms. R. was cognizant that many individuals were unaware of the community services available to them. It was this awareness combined with her own desire to become employed that prompted her to seek admission to the Older Advocate Project.

Ms. E., Mr. B., and Ms. R. were selected as case studies because they best illustrated how the training program served as a solution to individual role problems produced by their age situation. They had all been in the work force, they had contact with the aging population through their own work, they recognized the need to assist this population segment, yet they did not consider themselves to be approaching old age. Ms. E. denied this fact verbally, Mr. B. through dress and returning to college, Ms. R. by passing for a younger person and desiring to return to a work situation. Each entered the program to a large degree in order to facilitate their continued involvement in activities which helped to hide their aging from themselves and others.

Theoretical Approaches

There are many divergent philosophies held by gerontologists with regard to aging. Disengagement theory holds that there is a reciprocal withdrawal process between the individual and society, i.e., people tend to disengage from all contacts (work, social, family) that are no longer wholly satisfying to them (Brown, 1974; Cummings and Henry, 1961). Activity theory, on the other hand, correlates activities with attitudes and holds that as people get older they continue the same activities and maintain the same attitudes as in the middle years (Havighurst and Albrecht, 1953). The use of substitute activities becomes important as a mechanism for working through different developmental issues (Havighurst, Neugarten, and Tobin, 1968).

Yet another theory of successful aging is continuity theory. Through the process of socialization, an individual develops preferences, habits, commitments, and many other qualities which become a part of his or her personality. As one gets older one has the tendency to continue and maintain these same qualities. Unlike activity theory, continuity theory does not assume that once roles become lost they will be replaced. The implication of continuity theory is that there are many possible adaptations to aging rather than just a few (Atchley, 1972).

Each of the three major theories could be used in analyzing the case studies presented here. Disengagement theory explains Mr. B.'s view of his own retirement. He senses that society is disengaging from him and is fighting to avoid a reciprocal disengagement from society. Ms. E. has also continued her work role and Ms. R. is seeking to refill this role. Here, however, continuity theory better explains why the maintenance of prior roles gives meaning to these women's present life situations. Their function as contributing members of society receiving financial remuneration has been fully ensconced into their way of life. Activity theory helps explain all three case studies. These people have been active since their early years and it is an ingrained impulse to remain that way though they are now chronologically older.

Retirement is an issue in the life span that is associated with much anxiety and age denial. This situation was demonstrated by other older advocate trainees as well as the cases presented. Retirement does not have a positive connotation in our society. It is silently understood that workers are allowed to retire and receive the pensions they have earned to facilitate their removal from roles in which they are seen as incapable of continuing productively (Rose, 1965). Retirement is perceived as an instrument that is successfully used to remove those people considered useless by society (Brown, 1964; Rose and Miller, 1965). Reichard, Levison, and Peterson (1962) assert that "the retired man is not simply a man who is unemployed, or a man out of the labor force, but an old man."

It is this negative approach that prompts a person such as Mr. B. to justify his early retirement by explaining that in Civil Service one is able to retire at 55 years of age. Both Ms. E. and Ms. R. had worked many years. Ms. E. was again in the work force because her former position became open and her employer was unaware of her chronological age. It was her contention that if her employer had been aware of her 59 years she would not have been offered the job. According to Barron in *The Aging American*, this stand is sustained by the public (Barron, 1961).

The three people described in this chapter felt a strong need to remain active in the work force. Their involvement in the project enabled them to gain skills and credentials that would facilitate this by counteracting the stigma of age. Ms. E. continued to work and became so involved that there was no time for vacations. Mr. B. attended college on a full-time basis, remained active in a union, and became associated with a community agency. Ms. R. became very involved in senior citizen transportation. All were, therefore, able to continue the activities of their middle years a while longer and to forestall the pressures to adopt a different life-style because of their age alone.

Conclusions

All three of the cases studied described persons denying their age in some specific ways. It is important to examine the meaning of denial. Is it a denial of one's self as a person growing old or a denial of stereotypes of old age? These three people saw themselves not as obsolete persons, but as physically and mentally alert and capable of being productive. However, they perceived that society did not view their maturity in that positive light. Was it not society that had been implying to them that being old was bad? Through their involvement with the training project these three persons were able to effectively continue old roles and engage in new ones. Thus the project became a facilitator of solutions to individual role problems created by stereotyped social views of aging.

References

Atchley, R. C. *The Social Forces in Later Life.* Belmont, Cal.: Wadsworth, 1972.

Barron, M. L. *The Aging American.* New York: Crowell, 1961.

Brown, A. Satisfying relationships for the elderly and their patterns of disengagement. *The Gerontologist,* 1974, *14,* 258–262.

Brown, J. P. *Counseling with Senior Citizens.* New Jersey: Prentice-Hall, 1964.

Cummings, E., and Henry, W. *Growing Old: The Process of Disengagement.* New York: Basic Books, 1961.

Havighurst, R. Successful aging. *The Gerontologist,* 1961, *1,* 407.

Havighurst, R., and Albrecht, R. *Older People.* New York: Longmans, 1953.

Havighurst, R., Neugarten, B., and Tobin, S. Disengagement and patterns of aging. In B. L. Neugarten (ed.), *Middle Age and Aging.* Chicago: University of Chicago Press, 1968.

Reichard, S., Levison, F., and Peterson, P. *Aging and Personality.* New York: John Wiley and Sons, 1962.

Rose, A. Mental health of normal older people. In A. Rose and W. Peterson (eds.), *Older People and Their Social World.* Philadelphia: F. A. Davis, 1965.

Rose, A., and Miller, S. The social dilemma of the aging leisure participant. In A. Rose and W. Peterson (eds.), *Older People and Their Social World.* Philadelphia: F. A. Davis, 1965.

8

The Senior Companions: We Help Them and They Help Us

N. Claire Kowalski

The Senior Companion Program Nationally

Two needs of elderly persons recognized by the 1971 White House Conference on Aging are the need to perform useful roles and the need to live independently in the community as long as possible. Part of the response to these needs was the authorization of the Senior Companion Program under Action in October 1973.[1] During the following summer 18 Senior Companion projects were funded in 17 states. By the end of 1976 45 projects with a total of more than 1,600 volunteers were in operation throughout the country, each administered by a local public or private nonprofit agency. Senior Companions are low-income persons over 60 years of age who are no longer in the regular work force. They are employed 20 hours a week to serve as companions to adults within a variety of settings complementing rather than replacing services the clients are already receiving from regular staff.

The Senior Companion Program was established with the primary goal of making available a rewarding and useful role to low-income elders. The program does this by providing supports necessary to enable older persons to give volunteer services. Participants receive a nontaxable stipend, which is not considered income and therefore does not affect their eligibility for food stamps, Medicaid, Supplemental Security Income, or government-subsidized housing. Transportation is

The author wishes to thank Elizabeth McKenna Jutras, Chief of Special Services, Rhode Island Department of Elderly Affairs and formerly Director of the Senior Companion Program in Rhode Island, and the individual Senior Companions, without whose sharing this chapter could not have been written.

provided or remuneration given, and arrangements are made for the Companions to have a nutritious noontime meal. The program provides an annual physical examination as well as ongoing information about a variety of community resources and benefits for which volunteers may be eligible. Socializing with other Senior Companions at meetings, meals, and during the ride to and from work is an important "fringe benefit" for many Senior Companions who live alone.

A second major goal of the Senior Companion Program is to provide assistance to adults with special needs. For the most part these are elderly, dependent persons. Some who live alone are faced with social, economic, physical, and mental health problems which jeopardize their chances of remaining in the community. In these cases Senior Companions visit regularly, help with simple household tasks, and encourage their home companions to become active in the community.[2] Other Senior Companions serve in residential institutions, where they offer the ongoing, personal social relationships that institutionalized persons often lack. Senior Companions who work in an institutional setting can usually serve a greater number of clients than those who visit private homes. In all cases Senior Companions are concerned friends who visit regularly to listen and to help.

Before beginning work Senior Companions have about 40 hours of training. This provides orientation to the program and instruction in the general skills which will be needed. Information is provided about federal, state, and local programs, such as Social Security, medical plans, and activities. Sometimes Senior Companions visit the agencies where these services are given, so that if they later return as applicants, they return to a familiar setting. Listening and enabling skills may be discussed during training and practiced in role play or case presentation.

Senior Companions work out of a volunteer station within the community or institution where they serve. Supervision is provided by Senior Companion Program staff and by volunteer station staff according to agreements made before Senior Companions are placed. Some projects have trained more Senior Companions than can be placed immediately. In such instances, the unplaced Senior Companions serve as substitutes for those who are ill or on leave, thus assuring continuity of service.

Each project has an advisory council to assist and support the staff in planning, policy making, and decisions regarding program and personnel. In addition to Senior Companions, the advisory council membership is likely to include representatives of the sponsoring agency, the institutions where Senior Companions serve, the area agency on aging, and older people from the community.

There is considerable diversity among the Senior Companion projects throughout the country. Some are urban, some rural; the sponsoring agency may be public or private nonprofit; service may be rendered in private homes, day care centers, or institutions; Senior Companions may be together with other Senior Companions most of the day or may work alone. Companions assigned to elderly persons in their own homes may concentrate on visiting and helping with light housekeeping, while others assigned to elderly who live in a housing project may try to involve these people in activities at the project. Senior Companions in one residential setting may engage in social and recreational activities, and those in another may help feed and groom their companions. This means that, just as elderly persons themselves, each Senior Companion project develops its own individual character and no single model can be applied to all.

Who are the Senior Companions? Three-quarters are between 60 and 70 years of age but a few are over 80. About half are white and about a third black. Over three-quarters are female. The main motivation for being a Senior Companion is the desire to help others. The stipend and the opportunity to remain active are also important incentives.[3]

Who are the people served by Senior Companions? Most are similar in age to the Senior Companions, although a few are in their 50s. About half live in their own homes. The rest are seen in day care centers or residential institutions. The Senior Companions perceive their companions as being lonely and depressed, especially those who live in institutions. These are seen as needing companionship, while those in their own homes are more likely to need personal care and help with housekeeping. Whatever the situation, both Senior Companions and their supervisors believe that the Senior Companions are instrumental in helping their home and institutional companions become happier and more active. As a result of their association with Senior Companions they often become more willing or able to care for themselves and more outgoing.

The Senior Companion Program in Rhode Island

A grant received by the Division on Aging of the Rhode Island Department of Community Affairs paved the way for the first Rhode

Island Senior Companions to begin work in the fall of 1974. As a condition of the grant, Senior Companion volunteer stations had been prearranged. These were situated at both the Institute of Mental Health and the General Hospital of the Rhode Island Medical Center, at two geriatric day care centers, and at a community center. Referrals of persons in their own homes who could benefit from the services of Senior Companions were sought from the Department of Social and Rehabilitiative Services, Title III meal site projects, health centers, visiting nurse organizations, church and community action programs.

At first Rhode Island Senior Companions were recruited through newspaper advertising and senior community centers. Before long word of mouth brought more than enough volunteers. Some were put on a waiting list, others were referred to the Foster Grandparent Program or the Retired Senior Volunteer Program. As of March 1977, approximately 100 Rhode Islanders had taken the two weeks' training to become Senior Companions, had received program orientation, and had learned about community resources available to them and their companions.

The goal of training was for Senior Companions to achieve first the understanding and confidence to effect friendly and helpful relationships with their future companions, and second, some knowledge of techniques and resources. The processes of getting to know each other, sharing background information, and learning to accept each other's differences during the training period served as good practice for the relationships trainees later developed with their companions. Training served to bring to awareness the many positive elements of relating which trainees had practiced for years, and also other elements which can be detrimental to a helping relationship. Sessions included visits to geriatric wards for brief, but direct, experience in relating to elderly patients. At this point many Senior Companions were anxious about the task before them and how they would go about it. Together with supervisors they shared their initial reactions and considered ways of meeting the challenge. Evaluating relationship behavior modeled by supervisory staff and by trainees themselves was also effective. An earlier article by this author included discussion of training sessions held for the first two groups of Rhode Island Senior Companions and explicated concepts which trainees found useful in understanding the implications of their own on-the-job behavior (Kowalski, 1976).

During the first 2½ years of the project, 10 Senior Companions left because they and the program were not suited to each other, 3 died, and about 25 left because they moved from the area, took other employment, or developed health problems. One former Senior Companion whose personal situation deteriorated became a client of the program and began receiving home visits.

Rhode Island Senior Companions range in age from 60 to 85 (1977 figures). Twenty percent are male, 15 percent are black. One American Indian and one Asian are in the group, along with a number of persons of Italian, Portuguese, and French backgrounds. These latter bring at least one foreign language to their work and can relate especially well with companions of these tongues. For the most part Senior Companions have had relatively little formal education, have started work young, and have had modest income all their lives. Quite a number have personal experience of unemployment, welfare, and food stamps.

About 30 percent of the Senior Companions serve companions in their own homes. The rest are distributed between the Institute of Mental Health, the General Hospital, and two geriatric day care centers. Companion assignments are usually between members of the same sex.

The core of the Senior Companion Program is the ongoing, individual relationships between Senior Companions and their companions. For this reason substitutes are not assigned during temporary absences of Senior Companions. Sick or vacationing Senior Companions have sometimes communicated with their companions by mail or phone. At times, other Senior Companions serving at the same volunteer station have looked in on the companions who are alone.

Members of the program wear bar pins identifying them by name as Senior Companions. At the annual recognition banquet, those who have served for a year receive an attractive oval pin with the letters SCP. Occasionally an outing is planned for all Senior Companions together. They may be included individually in excursions organized by their volunteer stations. For a few, new horizons have opened through their association with volunteer station personnel.

Supervision is provided by three supervisors under the Senior Companion director and by volunteer station personnel. The Senior Companions working in institutions receive more constant supervision that those who visit individual homes. These latter tend to be independent, self-reliant persons who will call a supervisor if they have questions between meetings. They also have ties with a number of individuals and institutions in the community. They see relatives and friends regularly, and take part in various social and activity programs. Some are "senior power" advocates, and supervisory staff encourage such advocacy when they find it. Rhode Island Senior Companions who do home visiting tend to be flexible persons who are responsive to changing circumstances and who also know their own limits. They do not need ongoing direction, nor do they rely primarily on the Senior Companion Program to fulfill their social or nutritional needs. They do, however, need the program for employment, purposeful activity, and recognition. The Senior Companions who serve in group settings are those who function best when they have a readily available source of guidance. They are also the people for whom the opportunity to socialize with other Senior Companions is important. The unmarried men, and some of the women, depend on the noon meal eaten together for their main nourishment of the day. It is apparent that the individual who enjoys serving companions at home might not enjoy working in a group setting, and vice versa. A Senior Companion's personality and preferences are taken into account when assignments are made. In the very few cases where a switch in setting has appeared desirable, this has been effected with good results. Some Senior Companions serving at the Medical Center have commented that they would not want to visit in homes "and be alone so much." One Senior Companion who visits companions at home declared that she would find it depressing to serve at the Medical Center.

The Rhode Island Senior Companion Advisory Copuncil meets bimonthly. This council is composed of volunteer station representatives, program supervisory staff, and two Senior Companions elected by their peers. At first these latter representatives hesitated to speak out, but they have now become active participants. They also relay news of council meetings back to those who elected them.

Senior Companions Speak for Themselves

In reply to the question, "What does it mean to you to be a Senior Companion?" most of those in the program said that it gives them a way to help other people. "We help them [companions] and they help us" and "It's good for us and it's good for them" were typical replies. The Senior Companions are aware of interdependence between themselves and those they serve. Some stated clearly, and others implied, "I may be in their [companions] place some day." Many Senior Companions referred to the importance of having worthwhile activity. "I don't want to play bingo and gossip. They tried to get me to do that where I live"

was one comment. Another woman remarked, "The Lord has helped
me be well enough to get out and help other people." Some reported
that working as a Senior Companion keeps them from worrying about
their own problems, such as a family member with incurable illness.
One said, "I work here and I work at home. My husband isn't well and I
also take care of my mother who is 84. But it's good for me to get away
from them for a while each day and be here." One man summarized
what the program means to Senior Companions when he said, "It feels
good to know you're helping somebody."

None of the Senior Companions doubt the value of their work.
"They [companions] are happier because we're here," "They're sorry
when Friday comes because we won't be back until Monday," and
"When we get there they have the tables and chairs all ready waiting
for us," are typical comments. Many Senior Companions remarked on
positive changes they have seen in their companions. They attributed
these changes partly to their own efforts. "One man I visited with went
home from this hospital. He wanted to. That made me feel real good."
Or "She and I talk Italian. Before I came she hardly spoke to anyone."
And again, "I know she's eating better since I began visiting her, and
she looks better."

Some Senior Companions also noted changes in themselves since
they joined the program. "I had worked as a waitress. I wasn't used to
visiting people. I had to get used to it." "Now when I wake up I look
forward to the day, except Saturday and Sunday." "Our family wasn't
used to kissing," one lady said, "but the 89-year-old I visit, she likes to
kiss. She asked me to kiss her. So I thought, why not, and now I do."
another Senior Companion reported feeling better when she was
working and maintaining a routine.

When asked what parts of the program were important to them,
Senior Companions repeated the remarks reported above. None
mentioned the stipend, the noon meal, or transportation. Indeed, when
questioned further, some complained about the senior transportation
service. A few said that the stipend just covers expenses they incur
going to work every day. Whether they wish they could afford to serve
without remuneration, whether the stipend is considered a private
matter, or whether for some undetermined reason, most Senior
Companions avoided speaking of the stipend. As trainees, however,
several had indicated that the stipend would be a welcome addition to
their income. Perhaps the stipend, the noon meal, and transportation
are looked on as an integral part of the program rather than as
benefits.

Senior Companions spoke of various activities they undertake with their companions, often adding, "She knows I'm her friend." Those at the Medical Center told of having little initial success when they tried to introduce games on the wards. They said that at first they would relate with the most outgoing patients, or even talk among themselves, while patients who were unresponsive to their invitations observed from the sidelines. As time went by and the same Senior Companions appeared on the ward each weekday, greeting the withdrawn as well as the sociable patients, the former began to respond. A Senior Companion told of a companion whom she had difficulty engaging in conversation. "She would talk only a very little. So I told her my age and about myself. I didn't just ask her questions. We began exchanging information. Now we're friends." As Senior Companions walk through the long hospital corridors on their way to visit their companions, they also greet by name and have a cheery word for patients of all ages who live along these corridors. Some Senior Companions reported sadly that several patients with whom they worked had regressed, explaining, "It's their illness, you know, and they can't really help it." Sometimes Senior Companions play cards or other games with their companions at the Medical Center. Bingo is especially popular because prizes are given. In this setting Senior Companions initiate activities and relationships. At the daycare centers Senior Companions are likely to join their companions in programmed activities, helping them to achieve the activity goal and encouraging them by giving individual attention. Those serving in private homes bring the same friendship and individual concern as do Senior Companions in other settings. Depending on the needs and limitations of their companions, they may do shopping, bring mail and write letters, perform a few household tasks, help with food preparation, and accompany their companions to social activities or appointments outside home. One Senior Companion has continued to visit four companions with whom she was formerly involved at home. Each is presently in the local health center recovering from surgery or a broken bone. This adaptable Senior Companion commented on a companion, known to be a trying lady: "When she begins to gossip, I just say goodbye, see you tomorrow."

Answers to the question, "What would you be doing if you were not a Senior Companion?" ranged from "Just rocking and watching TV," "Feeling sorry for myself," and "Biting my fingernails," to "Babysitting for my grandchildren," "Working as a boiler engineer like I used to," and "Traveling. I've been in 20 states and 9 countries." Several referred to their former employment, then remarked that it would be too strenuous for them now. Others told how they had been required to retire before they wanted to because of age. One attractive and congenial lady told how she had let herself go into "bad shape" after retirement. She had inquired about the Senior Companion Program only because of the repeated insistence of a friend who saw how poorly she looked. An 84-year-old Senior Companion was looking forward to her forthcoming two-week trip to Florida, after which she would be returning to her Senior Companion work.

One lady summarized an important part of every Senior Companion's work. "I listen. Maybe it's the same story they told me yesterday, but I listen all over again today." She went on to describe the companions she serves at home. "These people grew up in big families. They are used to a lot of people around. Now they can't get out much. Their grandchildren and great-grandchildren don't visit like their sons and daughters used to, and they are lonely. We'll all be that way some day. Any one of us might be like that." Senior Companions in every setting echoed this last statement.

Discussion

The need to have sponsored volunteer programs for the elderly and the potential benefit of such programs for both community and participants has been documented (Filipic, Harel, and Schur, 1976), and there are manuals concerning the older volunteer (Ethel Percy Andrus Gerontology Center, 1976). The following discussion is specific to the Senior Companion Program, the benefits accruing from it to clients and volunteers, and some of the reasons for these benefits.

Originators of the Senior Companion Program knew that in order to realize the potential of older, low-income volunteers the program would have to include a number of enabling features. Hence the training, the ongoing supervisory support, the stipend, and the focus on the individual applicant in the selection of trainees. In our society there are very few opportunities for low-income persons over 60 to be considered for employment on the basis of their own potential. The Senior Companion Program includes some individuals over 80, some who have pacemakers, and many who would for one reason or another be considered unlikely employees elsewhere. Another of the program's enabling features is that it offers opportunity to serve in diverse settings, one of which may suit a volunteer better than another. The program is flexible enough so that neither volunteer nor client is required to fit rigid categories.

Health, as defined by the World Health Organization, is "a state of complete physical, mental and social well-being, and not merely the absence of disease or infirmity" (WHO, 1946). The Senior Companion Program has contributed to the threefold well-being of the people it employs. They in turn have reached out to those they serve, helping the companions to cope more effectively and to fulfill some of their physical, mental, and social needs. National figures from the first year of the program's operation indicate that Senior Companions contributed to preventing, delaying, or reversing institutionalization of over 500 companions. There is no documentation of the revitalizing effect the program has had on Senior Companions themselves or the extent to which participation has removed them from the number of potential institutional reidents. Undoubtedly, however, the Senior Companion Program has helped to improve the quality of life for all those it involves, clients and volunteers alike.

For Senior Companions the program has increased income, at least slightly, and promoted good health through a nutritious daily meal and an annual physical examination. It has also provided opportunities for social interaction with peers and has offered a meaningful work role which fosters positive self-identity. For companions the program has, at the very least, brought a new link to the world outside their place of residence, increased social activity, and provided a friend who is a potential confidante. Many companions have also received help with tasks they would not otherwise accomplish. None of this has decreased job opportunities for people in the regular work force. In other words, the Senior Companion Program has provided services that would not otherwise have been available to its clients.

The Senior Companion Program provides services to people who are elderly and below the level of good mental and physical health. Moreover, the volunteers are persons who themselves, because of age or physical or social limitations, could be candidates for the program's services in the not very distant future. In such circumstances the accomplishments of the Senior Companion Program can seem quite remarkable. The fact is, however, that the program has tapped human resources that are usually undervalued, i.e., the natural understanding and helping ability that elderly people can offer each other. The result is a program that provides services through nontraditional volunteers to a problem-prone population that is shunned by many success-oriented professionals. Monk and Cryns (1974) pointed out that the elderly who engage in traditional volunteer service tend to be affluent, well-educated individuals of relatively high social status. Many Senior Companions, to the contrary, have had little formal education. All currently have low income, either because they have always been part of the lower socioeconomic class, or because of downward mobility following widowhood, divorce, or retirement. Individual Senior Companions may themselves be receiving a variety of services.

Both volunteers and clients in the Senior Companion Program are of an age to experience what Butler (1975) has termed "ageism," i.e., society's negative prejudice toward the elderly. With advancing years both are suffering sensory loss and a variety of health problems. Both are losing friends and relatives through death. The Senior Companions who serve in homes usually live in the same neighborhoods as their companions. In short, the persons who deliver service differ relatively little from those who receive it. Probably it is this similarity that accounts for the great empathy between the volunteers and their clients. The benefits to the companions and the job satisfaction for the Senior Companions are also enhanced by the similarity between them. Companions may aspire and strive to cope as successfully as the Senior Companions who they perceive as people like themselves. They are likely to accept help and encouragement from someone with whom it is possible to identify, someone who is a sort of neighbor surrogate. Most Senior Companions have occupied the neighbor role for years, although they are likely to be new to the volunteer role. The phrase often used by Senior Companions, "this could be me," indicates the bonds based on perceived similarity that they feel with their companions. In this program volunteers and clients speak the same language, both literally and figuratively. Program staff have noted that the clients are likely to talk to and confide in other elders who they feel share and understand their problems. Senior Companions and their companions soon discover common experiences of locale, person, or event around which they can reminisce. This can be mutually beneficial because both are of the age when they are likely to be involved in the Life Review (Butler and Lewis, 1973). Sorting through memories together can help each to integrate elements of the life each has lived, and hopefully to find meaning in it.

Back (1976) has pointed out that because of declining fertility rates there will be an increasing number of persons without close relatives and that as a result the importance of one's generational role and relationships with age peers may increase. Such are the relationships within the Senior Companion Program. This author believes that it is both fitting and beneficial that all types of services for the elderly be planned, administered, and delivered by older persons. Young people who have a particular expertise that is not sufficiently available among the ranks of the elderly will continue to be employed. However, other things being equal, it must be recognized that elders bring to any work with their peers the added dimension of understanding achieved through their own experience of living and aging. This is the unique talent that the Senior Companion Program taps. This is the essence of the program in which "we help them and they help us."

Notes

1. Senior Companions are financed through a grant with ACTION under Title II of the Domestic Volunteers Services Act of 1973.
2. In this chapter, the individuals served by Senior Companions are referred to as "companions."
3. Data in this chapter that refer to the nationwide program are according to the Senior Companion Program Study by Booz, Allen and Hamilton, Inc.

References

Back, K. W. Personal characteristics and social behavior: Theory and method. In R. H. Binstock and E. Shanas (eds.), *Handbook of Aging and the Social Sciences*. New York: Van Nostrand Reinhold, 1976.

Booz, Allen and Hamilton, Inc. Produced for ACTION. *Senior Companion Program Study Phases I and II*. Washington, D.C., 1975.

Butler, R. N. *Why Survive? Being Old in America*. New York: Harper and Row, 1975.

Butler, R. N., and Lewis, M. I. *Aging and Mental Health*. Saint Louis: C. V. Mosby, 1973.

Ethel Percy Andrus Gerontology Center. *Releasing the Potential of the Older Volunteer* and *Older Volunteer Training Program*, 1976.

Filipic, L., Harel, Z., and Schur, D. The contribution of the retired senior volunteer program toward improving the well-being of its participants and their community. Paper presented at the 29th Annual Scientific Meeting of the Gerontological Society, New York, October 1976.

Kowalski, N. C. Smother love vs tough love. *Social Work*, 1976, *21*, 319–321.

Monk, A., and Cryns, A. G. Predictors of voluntaristic intent among the aged: An area study. *The Gerontologist*, 1974, *14*, 425–429.

White House Conference on Aging. *Toward a National Policy on Aging*, Vol. 2. Washington, D.C.: U.S. Gov. Printing Office, 1972.
World Health Organization. *Constitution of the World Health Organization*. Public Health Report 61, 1946, 1268–1277.

9

The Limitations of a Volunteer Cohort Group for the Elderly

Elizabeth Bristowe

Elderly Volunteers in Developed Nations

The United Nations considers any country to be "old" if more than 8 percent of the population is over 65.[1] By this definition, Canada entered the "family" of old nations in 1971 (Science Council of Canada, 1976). In 1966 in this country there were approximately 1.5 million persons over the age of 65, almost five times the 1901 total. The population aged 75 and over has increased nearly six times since 1901, and it is estimated that the present numbers will increase two and one-half times by 1991 (Special Committee of the Senate on Aging, 1966). In common with the rest of the developed world, Canada is experiencing not only the increased age of elderly individuals but also the aging of the population itself (Beckman, 1976).

British Columbia is the western province of Canada and has a population of 2.25 million people, with the third largest share of Canada's elderly. An analysis of census data indicates that the proportion of elderly immigrants to the province is high (Mercer, 1977), probably because of the climate and favorable estate-duty legislation. This elderly migration stream can be expected to continue and may result in an even more substantial increase in the elderly population. These trends hold great significance for social planning since the elderly are the fastest growing major demographic component of Canadian society.

Escalating costs, as well as demands, require that governments continue to explore new ways of ensuring that the programs they mandate are actually delivered to the population for whom they are planned. Increasing attention is being paid to the fact that the acceptance of these services are often issues quite separate from their provision. Money and personnel alone cannot solve the problem of nonparticipation in social programs by the elderly. While their needs may be great, people at risk are often unwilling to see a welfare service as an acceptable alternative to discomfort (*Perception*, 1978). "Old people often cling to their isolation not because they do not need help but because they are afraid of the form it will take" (Age Concern, 1974). While there will always be economic restraints on the services that can be made available, these do not have to inhibit the use of imagination or the quality of caring shown either by social administrators, paid casework staff, or volunteers.

Voluntary work has always been an attribute of the Western way of life and social planners are starting to take advantage of it. Although voluntarism declined somewhat in the first half of the twentieth century (perhaps due to the increasing professionalization of the human services), it has recently been regaining momentum and is now being incorporated into the formal structure of many public programs to fill the gaps in service delivery (Monk and Cryns, 1974). Many attempts have been made in Canada, as elsewhere, to develop voluntary lateral support systems for people who are broadly defined as being at risk. The impetus may come from professionals, from volunteers, or from the people in need. Very frail institutionalized elderly or old persons living alone and going through an almost imperceptible process of "unraveling" in the community are often seen as target groups for senior volunteer programs. One frequently adopted approach to meeting their needs is the setting up of like-to-like or cohort groupings, which have had great success in other areas. It will be suggested here, however, that although this model will continue to be effective in many forms of intervention, it is not always appropriate for the elderly volunteer.

Reasons for volunteering are numerous. In a study carried out in 30 Canadian cities, "to help others" and "to feel useful and needed" were the chief reasons for volunteering in the 60+ age group (Anderson and Moore, 1975). The expectation among the elderly is high, therefore, that volunteering will tend to sustain well-being and avoid some of the self-fulfilling prophecies of decremental change with aging. These expectations will best be realized when the needs of both the volunteer and the client are recognized in appropriate ways. When this is not done at the outset, one or the other will fail to benefit.

The Senior Citizens Counselors Program

The Senior Citizens Counselors of British Columbia is an example of a volunteer program introduced by a government in an attempt to improve service delivery. The stated goal of the program is to "provide a service whereby active, knowledgeable, community-minded senior citizens serve as resource people to assist other senior citizens."[2]

The program was started in 1967 by the provincial government. It was becoming increasingly clear that the workings of bureaucracy often prevented older people from receiving the services for which they were eligible. An advocacy system was envisaged in which able retired people would act as problem solvers. Initially, 15 persons, all elderly, were selected to form a pilot project. Next, local groups of old age pensioners and seniors organizations throughout the province were approached and 25 volunteers were appointed to work under the auspices of the local government welfare offices to determine the needs of older persons in their communities. A questionnaire approach was used and the main areas of concern were identified as housing, medical services (hearing aids, glasses, and ambulances), legal advice, difficulties understanding the ramifications of income tax returns, allowance and pension forms, residential care, and the provision of drop-in social centers. Conference and workshop training sessions started in October 1968, for 40 people. Fifty-three counselors went to the first Conference in 1969, and in 1971 there were 60 participants throughout the province.

A counselor is described as a volunteer worker, appointed by the provincial government to aid older persons with their problems: someone in their own age bracket, living in their area to whom they can turn for assistance knowing that their right to confidentiality will be respected. They are appointed by the minister of human resources, and receive an enamel pin, calling cards, report and journal forms, and an information kit containing pamphlets on a wide range of services available to older persons. Many counselors work out of existing senior drop-in centers where in some instances they have been provided with permanent office space.

The chief role of the counselor is to put people in contact with agencies or persons who can meet their particular needs. More specifically, the services provided include helping clients to complete forms, making referrals to appropriate community agencies for assistance, answering questions about government programs, helping to organize community events, providing assistance with transportation and accommodation, and providing friendly visiting. The counselor should be active in the community, be knowledgeable, have organizational ability, and have a special interest in and understanding of the particular needs and problems of the aged.[3]

The numbers of calls and interviews counselors make during a month varies from 20 to 150. Transportation to doctors offices and hospitals is now a considerable part of their work, especially in the north where there is no public transit service and a trip to a hospital may mean a round trip journey of 120 miles. Older persons in these isolated areas are independent and inclined only to ask for help in an emergency. Consequently, the type of service requested and provided is entirely different from the friendly visiting described by counselors in the suburbs. One report submitted from a remote part of the province lists, without comment, washing the feet of an old timer, giving him an enema, washing his dishes, and cleaning up his dirty shack as among the services provided during the month.

Some ongoing training is given through regional workshops which continue to be a useful part of the program. They provide an opportunity for counselors to gain clarification of new government programs as well as the chance to meet representatives from the various ministries and compare problems and solutions with each other. The program is seen as particularly effective in regions where social workers and volunteers cooperate. The whole area of the attitude of paid staff to volunteers is important in any program and will repay further study. Unfortunately, the remark, "Well, if what they are doing is worth anything, they'll be paid for it won't they?" is not uncommon. While it certainly says more about the speaker than about the program, it also points up the necessity for continuing reevaluation of their own attitudes by professionals and of the quality of their service by volunteers.

According to the provincial coordinator of the program, social workers also benefit personally from the workshops even though their own perception of their role is primarily that of "resource people." She comments, "These workshops are good for staff. They see seniors there as regular people, not just as old folks who need help."[4]

An Evaluation of the Program

In January 1978 there were 114 Senior Citizens Counselors who responded primarily to requests for information, transportation, and form completion. The only material available on which to base an evaluation of the program comes from the monthly report, which was designed initially as an application for reimbursement of expenses of up to $60. These data should be interpreted with care because although the form used is itself standardized, its use by the senior counselors themselves is not.

The counselor report form asks for information about the number of contacts, personal and telephone, made in the following areas: income maintenance, health services, maintaining family relationships, living accommodation, home-delivered meals, home aides, friendly visiting, legal aid, transportation, and miscellaneous.

A survey of reports submitted during 1977 shows that the filling in of various forms was the biggest single presenting problem. (The magnitude of this difficulty is emphasized by the variations in the ways in which counselors themselves complete their own claims. The limited reliability of data from counselor report forms became clear when it was realized that a number of them listed all interactions in multiples of 5.) Forms with which clients need assistance, all of which are engendered by different levels of government, can be divided into two categories: demand forms, which must be completed to avoid penalty, and supply forms, which initiate a service to an individual if the request is made in the right way. The elderly feel under pressure to complete the demand forms, such as income tax returns, and this is reflected seasonally in requests for help made to counselors. Supply forms often refer to new services which may be poorly understood and are not used to advantage unless the counselors themselves initiate the process in their own communites.

The mode of response chosen by individual counselors to requests for assistance is interesting in that it appears to be consistent over time. The reports tend always to show a preponderance of phone calls over interviews or vice versa. Whether this is due to lack of transportation, differences in reporting procedures, or personality characteristics of the counselor which result in a filtering process is not known. It does seem that the type of contact reflects the counselor's preretirement background, e.g., "legal aid" was the service noted most frequently by a man with legal training. It is not clear, however, whether this is due to the reporting system he used or whether he is known in his community for offering this kind of help.

The category "friendly visiting," which may include visiting the sick, is reported infrequently suggesting that there may be little tolerance of the frail elderly. It is also entirely possible that the frail elderly themselves may not want to be visited by other old people.

The category "miscellaneous" covered over 50 percent of the calls made. With laudable economy of words, one counselor's sole monthly comment was that he had encountered "problems too numerous to relate."

In summary, two conclusions emerge from analysis of the limited data available. First, although the initial range of program objectives was wide, including both information giving and personal support, informal evaluation indicates that a selection process occurs by which the counselors tend to limit their involvement to task-oriented situations. It is suggested that although some of the counselors' own needs are being met in this way, the need of the frailer elderly for warm personal contacts is at times overlooked. Second, in discussing any project such as this it is important to stress the personal qualities and goals of each counselor. The data suggest that the informal structure of the program leaves it largely up to the individual to develop his or her own style of service. Counselors' service patterns vary from on-call, 24-hour availability to a very limited telephone contact confined to information giving only. As Faulkner (1975) points out, "individuals who prefer person to person rather than group volunteering have different personality characteristics" and a great deal of work remains to be done in this area to maximize the benefits of volunteering, both to volunteers themselves and to the community.

Implications

In *Future Shock*, Toffler (1971) sees the time as almost upon us when in order to meet the needs of society, large numbers of persons in the community will be deputized to listen to other lay persons. In return, he comments, "they will have access to others for similar assistance in the course of their own adaptive development" (p. 387). Indeed, in her inaugural address as President of the American Psychological Association in Janaury 1974, Dr. Leona Tyler emphasized that the role of the professional in direct services is becoming increasingly limited, except in crisis intervention. The purely logistical difficulty of too few trained workers combined with the realization that nonprofessional, prepared lay persons work at least as effectively with their peers as professional staff are undoubtedly contributing factors here (e.g., Truax and Lister, 1970).

In a national survey taken in Britain among 2,700 people of pensionable age, Age Concern found that 56 percent of the elderly felt that no one relied on them. It is pointed out that "not being relied on" by anyone can be an important factor in the poor health, loneliness, social isolation complex of problems of the aged (Age Concern, 1974). The expectation that older persons are anxious to be active and involved appears to be almost a worldwide phenomenon. Providing opportunities to be of assistance to their peers is one obvious way of counteracting the sense of role loss among the aged.

Even among decision makers who recognize the importance of older persons' contributions, stereotypic thinking may restrict the range of elderly who are allowed involvement. For example, the Government of British Columbia suggests that Senior Citizens Counselors should be elderly themselves and be knowledgeable about their own community and the service that it offers. Further requirements are that they be active in the community, be involved in community organizations, and be physcially able to get out. Questions can be raised on these latter points since a most valuable role can be filled by a person who, although bedfast, is mentally alert and who spends time on the telephone maintaining contact and service linkage. Carkhuff (1968) indicated that counselors, professional and lay, do tend to select for treatment and continue in treatment, people who are much like themselves in demographic descriptions. Such suggestions need to be borne in mind in order to maximize the benefits to both the helpers and the helped.

On the other hand, older persons often express their dislike of spending time with "all those old people" and the experience of this project has suggested that interaction with frail elderly tends to be avoided by older volunteers. Peer counseling among the aged may be significantly different in at least one respect from groups like, for example, Alcoholics Anonymous (AA). In AA the counselors can see in the client what they once were and can congratulate themselves on no longer being in the same plight. For the elderly, the situation is reversed, with the counselors reminded constantly of what they may become.

If active old people are asked to volunteer to spend their time with frail and dependent elderly, the program may work to their mutual disadvantage unless great sensitivity is shown by the program director to the needs of all people involved. Wise selection of aged volunteers and the clients to whom they are assigned will help to ensure that the benefits are mutual. Additionally, training and support groups are important for all volunteers. For older people who have expressed a particular interest in work with the frail elderly (and no other older person should be expected to be so involved), they are essential.

The need for service in the community on a one-to-one basis exists and will undoubtedly expand, particularly among older persons. How that need can be met in ways that contribute to the well-being of all the people concerned requires careful consideration. It may well be that rather than insisting on the use of the model of the self-help group, it will be found to be more appropriate to deliberately move in the opposite direction. In British Columbia, Senior Citizen Counselors could be redefined as older volunteers who are involved specifically in, for example, work with younger mentally or physically handicapped adults. Younger adults in turn should be encouraged to form information and support groups for the aged. Where projects have been initiated along these lines the success rate in terms of personal satisfaction appears to be high. It may well be that, in relation to older persons, the usefulness of the self-help concept is limited and social planners should take time to pause and reconsider the direction in which they are headed.

Planning for volunteer participation must also take into account the sorts of people who will be able to carry out the programs in the foreseeable future. Today's older persons have been influenced by a work-dominated society in which they were accustomed to definition largely in terms of their jobs, not by what they did in their spare time. For people who raised families in the depression the implications of being without work are reflected in the desperation with which many of them face retirement, the difficulty they may have in asking for help when they need it, and the type of service they are willing to offer. Typically, the elderly person who is interested in volunteering today tends to be younger and better educated than someone who does not want to be involved (Monk and Cryns, 1974). Since people retiring in the next quarter of a century will as a group leave the work force with a higher level of education than any of their forebears, both their interest in volunteer work and their expectation of personal satisfaction from it can be expected to increase. Cutler (1976) comments on "trends which suggest that future cohorts of older persons may belong to and participate in voluntary associations to a greater extent than current cohorts of the elderly." An obvious extension of the finding that individual volunteer style is a mjaor program outcome variable is the ncessity of considering changing cohort trends in planning for the continuance of volunteer programs.

In short, in discussing any volunteer program, it is overly simplistic to present it as merely the delivery of a service to those defined as clients. The concept of intracohort self-help groups among older persons has at least as much significance for the provider of service as for the recipient. The implications of such programs for the elderly helpers requires further examination.

Notes

1. Age 65 is taken throughout this chapter as conventionally marking the beginning of old age, although it is viewed as less than satisfactory. It ignores both the differences between individuals of the same chronological age and the categories of young-old, middle-old, and old-old.
2. Material provided by the Ministry of Human Resources, Victoria, B.C., 1977, in a "kit" given to Senior Citizen Counselors.
3. From an undated circular distributed by the Ministry of Human Resources, Victoria, B.C.
4. In a personal interview with the author in Victoria, B.C., 1978.

References

Age Concern. Manifesto Series. London, 1974.
Beckman, A. C. The aging of the population. Third Annual Easton-McCarney Memorial Lecture, Wilfred Laurier University, Ontario, November 1976.
Carkhuff, R. R. Differential functioning of lay and professional helpers. *Journal of Counseling Psychology*, 1968, *15*, 117–126.
Cutler, S. Age profiles of membership in sixteen types of voluntary associations. *Journal of Gerontology*, 1976, *31*, 462–470.
Faulkner, A. O. The black aged as good neighbors. *The Gerontologist*, 1975, *15*, 554–559.

Mercer, J. Demographic trends and the location of older people. Paper presented at a workshop on Housing and Care for Older People, University of British Columbia, May 10, 1977.

Monk, A., and Cryns, A. G. Predictors of voluntaristic intent among the aged. *The Gerontologist,* 1974, *14,* 425–429.

Perception. Editorial Comment on the Elderly, January/February 1978, p. 36.

Science Council of Canada. *Implications of the Changing Age Structure of the Canadian Population.* Ottawa, June 1976.

Special Committee of the Senate on Aging. Report, 1966.

Toffler, A. *Future Shock.* Toronto: Bantam Books, 1971.

Truax, C. B., and Lister, J. L. Effectiveness of counselors and counselor aides. *Journal of Counseling Psychology,* 1970, *17,* 331–334.

Part IV
The State of the Art

10

Current Knowledge and Questions Regarding the Use of Older Workers in Mental Health Systems: The State of the Art

Rosemary McCaslin

The programs sampled in the preceding chapters indicate the wide range of roles that older workers have filled and continue to fill in mental health systems. Increased attention is being given to the potential uses of older workers in general and a fair amount of research has been done on the issues involved. In many cases, the older workers whose performances have been examined have been engaged in tasks that are supportive of the mental health needs of other people. Yet there has been little systematic attention to the benefits of utilizing older workers directly in the mental health system.

The revised Mental Health Systems Act (P.L. 96-536) gave priority to services for older people and other underserved groups. At the same time, it allowed funds to go to small, community-based projects in addition to community mental health centers. Since these funds were subsequently placed in block grants with other programs, the emphasis on diverse, locally defined service delivery models should be even stronger. Under these conditions, it should be possible to develop creative programs which draw on the unique contributions that older persons can make to the system and its clients. At the same time, such programs could enhance and maintain the mental health of the older persons they employ. Such programmatic thrusts would surely be in keeping with the spirit of the report of the President's Commission on Mental Health (1978), which spurred the new public law as that report emphasized the embeddedness of mental health problems in the social environment.

Of course, the funds available for such mental health programs may be severely curtailed in coming years if the currently ascendant philosophy of government austerity continues to hold sway. It is also possible that, if mental health funds become part of block grants, they will have to compete directly with other interests for their funding. Under either or both of these conditions, mental health programs will need to present the most economically efficient plans possible for meeting public needs. For this reason, too, the use of older workers seems a productive strategy. Older workers are often concerned that their earned income does not exceed Social Security limits and thus are willing to work for relatively lower wages than younger persons. The contributions that can be derived from these highly experienced workers, therefore, often come quite cheaply. Furthermore, the argument that employment of older persons is supportive of their own mental health is even more important when the cost-benefit ratio of a proposed service strategy is in the forefront.

The time is right for serious examination of the potential usefulness of older workers to mental health programs. Not only is this approach enabled by current legislation, but it is also made more attractive by economic realities. Sufficient evidence exists regarding the benefits of such jobs to both the older workers and their clients that many of the costs and advantages of using these workers can be anticipated in advance. This chapter will review the most important thinking and data on older workers in the hopes that it can then be more readily drawn upon to support the development of new programs.

Contributions of Older Workers to Mental Health Programs

Studies of older workers in a variety of settings have consistently found them to be valuable additions to the staff. Typical is a study by Braver and Bowers (1977) which is one of the most extensive works to date on the actual experience of older workers and their colleagues. Looking at older persons employed under the federal Job Opportunities Program (P.L. 93-567), they obtained data from group interviews with 811 elderly employees and from questionnaires filled out by 518 individual supervisors and 463 agency directors. The job performance of the older workers was rated very high by their superiors: 50 percent were felt to be excellent employees and 31 percent to be good. Among those qualities identified as valuable in the older workers were a pride in their work that made for a very high quality of effort; dedication to the program; tactfulness, understanding of other people, dependability, and trustworthiness; and a combination of experience, skill, wisdom, and good judgment that made for workers who were prompt, conscientious, courteous, and cooperative.

A group of workers described in such glowing terms would certainly be a valuable addition to any agency or office. The question of interest is, in what ways can and should these attributes be put to use in mental health programs? The literature suggests that there are several appropriate answers.

Linkage Functions

A general approach to assessing the usefulness of older workers in mental health systems may be drawn from the "balance theory of coordination between bureaucracy and primary groups" developed by Litwak (1978).[1] In this view, bureaucratic institutions (such as a mental health center) are seen as being best equipped to deal with uniform tasks in which technical expertise can be predictably and systematically applied to achieve a desired result. Major uniform tasks in the mental health system would include psychotherapy, administration of psychotropic drugs, and behavioral programming in institutional settings. On the other hand, nonuniform tasks that involve "idiosyncratic influences, many contingencies, or frontier areas" are best handled by primary groups such as the family or neighborhood networks. Examples of these would be the teaching of daily living skills and appropriate social behavior and ongoing feedback on and support for healthy functioning. The events which make up human lives are seen as falling on a continuum of uniformity with both more and less uniform tasks required at different points in time.

The report of the most recent President's Commission on Mental Health (1978) generally concludes that the mental health system has succeeded fairly well in making uniform services available to its clients but is greatly lacking in its ability to provide for those nonuniform tasks which are also necessary to the support of the mentally ill. For example, they assert:

As a consequence of deinstitutionalization and the move to community care it is now being realized that to be maintained outside the hospitals, patients need a great many services that the mental health system itself is not equipped to give. There is increasing emphasis on the need for generic workers or case managers who can perform this integrating function.

It is hardly surprising that the gaps found in the mental health system would be on the nonuniform end of the continuum. Funding emphasis has largely been placed on provision of highly technical expertise by professionals such as psychiatrists, psychologists, and nurses. The most uniform tasks have been taken care of and it is now time to fill in the less uniform services which are no less important. Toward this end the President's Commission recommends that a major effort be developed in the area of personal and community supports which will

1. Recognize and strengthen the natural networks to which people belong and on which they depend
2. Identify the potential social support that formal institutions within communities can provide
3. Improve the linkages between community support networks and formal mental health services, and
4. Initiate research to increase our knowledge of informal and formal community support systems and networks

These recommendations are in line with Litwak's notion that a proper balance of distance must be maintained between the bureaucracy and the community if their relationship is to be harmonious and effective. It is not sufficient to simply assign uniform tasks to the agency and reserve nonuniform tasks for the family. Mental health patients are embedded in both of these systems and their problems may require the combined resources of the two systems for their resolution. Thus, the issue becomes how the agency and the community can be most effectively linked and their tasks coordinated.

Litwak suggests several ways in which the agency can reach out to effect linkages with the community, one of which is the use of *common messengers* or indigenous people to provide leadership in the interchange. He further suggests that these common messengers may be of three types: (1) the high-powered lay person (e.g., a nonprofessional agency board member), (2) the low-powered indigenous person (e.g., a paraprofessional case aide), or (3) the high-powered indigenous expert (e.g., a paid professional social worker who lives in the neighborhood). Each of these is seen as being most effective in a specific type of situation with all being potentially necessary to a continuing effective interface between agency and community.

Certainly, older workers can and do fill all three of the messenger roles in mental health systems. In this volume, Tristan and Bakke's grandparent advocates were high-powered lay persons in their communities who served a brokerage function between the Children and Youth Program and the local citizenry. McCaslin and Wilson underscore the importance of Senior Information and Outreach Service's paraprofessional older workers being lifelong residents of the communities in which they were providing services to clients. And Blumensohn's senior counselors were professionals who continued to put their expertise to work following retirement.

So, at the broadest level, it can be argued that older workers can be useful to mental health systems in a variety of ways that involve serving as common messengers linking the agency with the community. These are the major roles which must be added to the mental health system if its effectiveness is to be increased. Persons are needed who can represent the bureaucracy flexibly, allowing it to assess and at times intervene in nonuniform life events for which traditional professional expertise is not especially helpful.

It is often appropriate for the mental health system to have some involvement in nonuniform events in the lives of the chronically mentally ill, for example. Not only may a mixture of professional and nonprofessional assistance be required, but there are often no family and few friends at hand to supply the nonprofessional supports required by mental patients. Both before the fact, when agency policy is being decided, and during the event, when informal assistance with ties to the formal system is required, common messengers are needed to effect a meaningful partnership between agency professionals and community residents (both patients and nonpatients).

It can also be argued that older persons may be among the best choices to fill these linkage roles. The very stereotyping which reduces the elderly to "only" grandparents may work to their advantage, giving them access to parts of people's lives where professionals would not be welcomed. A surrogate grandparent may be more appropriate for a person needing support with a nonuniform task, such as learning to manage a household alone, than would the intervention of a professional. The latter runs the risk of underscoring the pathology which still exists rather than building up the areas of healthy functioning. The humanizing functions which older workers can add to mental health systems are mentioned often in the literature (e.g., Bowles, 1976;

Seguin, 1976; Thursz and Vigilante, 1978). Older persons are seen as being able to bring services closer to the consumer on a psychological level; because they are viewed as "human" rather than "professional," the distance between client and helper is lessened. Kent (1971) argued that such a humanizing of services is especially important for minority clients. He felt that minorities would be much better served by the use of indigenous workers to coordinate, expedite, and advocate for services for poor elderly and to hook up formal services with the informal network rather than being served by professional services sent to them from the top of the hierarchy.

It has also been suggested that older workers may be uniquely suited for these linkage roles because their presence tends to facilitate change. Meyer (1967) anticipated that the use of paraprofessionals in general in social service agencies might lead to professionals' reexamining their practice and developing new models of service as a result. Additionally, many programs have found that the use of older workers in established roles is useful in freeing other staff to give more time to their most critical services and/or to expand service into new areas (e.g., Bowles, 1976). In fact, Braver and Bowers (1977) found that the staff of agencies that had employed older workers had been able to develop new ways of reaching the community for both of these reasons. Two-thirds (66.1 percent) had been able to expand their services by handling more clients, staying open longer hours, etc., and 35.7 percent had been able to initiate new types of services. The majority (85 percent) felt that the agency would be unable to maintain this new level of service if it lost its older workers. Agency staff felt they had been able to give more attention to their clients and to serve more clients since older workers had been added to the staff. At the same time, they perceived an improvement in the quality of the agency's services stemming directly from the quality of the performance of the older workers and felt that an ongoing decline in service quality had been stopped by the alleviation of chronic staff shortages. What seems to be involved is a combination of increased personnel freeing professionals for creative examination of their services and an unsettling of old patterns as a result of nontraditional employees arriving on the scene.

It has also been noted that older workers often serve as pace setters in creating new service roles. They are not only willing to pioneer new ways of approaching problems but may also bring a new style to established roles that models productive changes in them (Bowles, 1976; Seguin, 1976). Sieder (1977) suggests that older workers may contribute directly to changing service patterns because they are more free than anyone else in the agency (or society) to push for change. Again, the negative stereotypes with which older persons have to contend may be used to their advantage. If one is a marginal person in society, one has less to lose and that position can be used as a motivating force to effect change both for selfish and for humanitarian reasons.

Unique Inputs: Direct and Indirect

It is clear that older workers can be (and have been) used to expand the services provided by agencies both directly and indirectly. Most of the projects described in this volume utilized older persons to create services that had not previously been provided in the community, or at least not by the sponsoring agency. Older workers have also proved especially useful in the provision of intensive one-to-one services for which existing staff do not have time. The Foster Grandparent Program might be considered the prototype of such programs in this country. The success of that program in providing individualized attention to institutionalized children has been widely reported. In a similar vein, Carter (1964) describes a program in which men from a senior center were recruited to meet weekly with small groups of underachievers, using their knowledge of life to connect what the children were learning in school to issues in the real world. They also met with teachers, principals, and parents so that their input would be integrated with the rest of the children's experience. The results of a blind evaluation showed that those who had received this extra input improved in school attendance, attitudes toward reading, confidence in using their skills, and enjoyment of school. This program seems a good example of the unique contributions that can be made by older persons: the teachers and other professionals in the school system would have been hard pressed to allocate the time that was spent by these older men and neither professionals nor parents were likely to have the store of life experience from which these men drew to reach the children.

From a somewhat different perspective it has been pointed out that the use of volunteers in an agency may have the effect of hiding the need for funding of professional services (e.g., Westerman, 1974). High-quality assistance added to a troubled agency may temporarily alleviate difficulties just enough that the ultimately necessary solution is put off until the situation grows even more serious.

The public relations benefits of hiring older workers is frequently mentioned in the literature (e.g., Braver and Bowers, 1977; Seguin, 1976). With the community at large, the presence of older workers in a program tends to legitimize the service by suggesting that the staff has a balanced and appropriately respectful view of both the assets and liabilities of old age. Additionally, older workers may be seen as particularly trustworthy by potential clients, especially by older persons with little experience with formal service systems. As McCaslin and Wilson point out, a peer may have more freedom to confront clients on their behavior and may be seen by the client as operating from a sounder knowledge base when they do so.

It has also been argued that because of the benefits that the older workers themselves derive from the experience (which will be discussed in the following section), the agency may be able to reduce some of its services to older people (Comfort, 1976; Rosenblatt, 1966). The program reported in this volume by Diamond, Brown, and Estes is a good example of the use of work or volunteer opportunities as a direct mental health service for older people, in place of or in addition to more traditional forms of assistance. Pearl (1964) has identified the factors that account for benefits accruing to the person in the helping role as including (1) an increased sense of power over his or her own life, (2) a tendency to begin to assess and resolve his or her own problems, and (3) a feeling of social usefulness and worth. These are certainly life changes that should have a positive effect on the overall mental health of the helper—in some cases a greater effect than could be derived from psychotherapeutic treatment. Additionally, there is reason to think that continued work activity may contribute to better physical health (Palmore, 1970), thus reducing the need for health-related services. The extra income gained through employment should reduce the need for direct and indirect financial assistance. It has even been suggested that older workers may indirectly affect the well-being of other older persons by serving as role models, which helps to debunk the negative stereotypes of old age which are too often internalized (Bowles, 1976).

Streib and Streib (1978) pointed out that older persons can and do make contributions to (1) their primary group, (2) the neighborhood or community, and (3) the larger society. They assert that the task is to prove that elderly who have not previously been involved directly in service in the latter two areas can be involved in such tasks in later life. The evidence is that communities and the society at large have much to gain from facilitating the involvement of older workers in mental health systems.

Contributions to Older Workers by Mental Health Programs

Evidence is increasing to validate our social beliefs regarding the value of meaningful work for people of all ages. For the elderly, who tend to have more underlying physical frailties than younger persons, the benefits of working are apparent at even the most basic level of health and longevity. Additionally, studies have found employed or otherwise active older persons to have better mental health, morale, and life satisfaction. Given the central place of work in our culture, it is hardly surprising that a person's work role should have such wide-ranging effects on his or her well-being. The issue of forced retirement is a major one that deserves increased attention from gerontologists.

Physical and Mental Health

The most basic level of well-being for an older person is the continuation of life and the maintenance of a reasonable degree of health and vigor. The presence or absence of meaningful work experiences appears to have an impact in this regard, although the cause and effect relation of the issues is at times cloudy.

The Duke Longitudinal Study (Palmore, 1970), for example, found work satisfaction to be the third highest predictor of longevity for men, following actuarial life expectancy and physical functioning. The correlation between work satisfaction and longevity alone was .19 and the three variables together explained 97 percent of the variance in longevity. It is often reported that health problems is a major reason that people retire, which suggests that the inability to work is an outgrowth of ill health. In other words, it is assumed that health problems cause both retirement and early death. While this is no doubt true in some cases, the Duke study's findings suggest that, at least for those healthy enough to continue working, positive work experiences also make a direct contribution to longevity and health.

Some work has been done to further specify the conditions under which the continuation of employment has an effect on longevity. Solem (1978) reports on a longitudinal study of 315 wage earners followed from just prior to retirement to four to five years after retirement. He found that persons who were at a higher risk of postretirement mortality if they were not working in some other capacity included older, single men; blue-collar workers; those in poor health; those who were forced to retire; those with poor communication with their children or with little contact with relatives or friends; and those having no membership in associations. He stresses the importance of social contact in the work setting. Of those who valued the social contact derived from working, 30 percent died within the first five years after retirement.

Other studies have found better physical and mental health among employees and volunteers. Seguin (1976), for example, reports that the older volunteers in a program sponsored by the Andrus Center were in better health as a result of increased physical activity and the presence of a daily schedule, and were in better mental health due to having increased contacts with other people and opportunities for worthwhile activity. The Special Task Force on Work in America (no date) noted that a major risk factor in heart disease is lack of congruence between job status and other life aspects, that unemployment is correlated with suicide, and that mental health is correlated with job satisfaction.

It would be overstating the case to say that work creates good health for older people. However, it appears that meaningful work can at least contribute to the maintenance of good health in the elderly. Further, available data suggest that work plays an especially important role in the lives of elderly with few social contacts from other sources. Such people are also at high risk for the sort of problems with which the mental health system deals. The employment of older workers, then, appears to make sense as a preventive health and mental health strategy.

Looking more closely at the mental health dimension, a number of studies have shown work to be related to measures such as morale and life satisfaction for elderly people. Crown (1977) reports that working old people are almost always found to score high on morale measures. Wylie (1970) found that the life satisfaction scores of older people increased after they had been involved in working with young people. Gray and Kasteler (1970) reported that foster grandparents had significant improvement in morale scores after participation in the program. Bradburn and Caplovitz's (1966) work indicated that people who are working are better adjusted than those who are not, and among those who are not working, those with high degrees of social participation are the better adjusted. The Duke studies (Palmore, 1970) showed activity level to be correlated with satisfaction with various aspects of life among older people.

Attitude measures such as morale and life satisfaction can serve as global indicators of mental health. Since several aspects of the experience of workng may affect these subjective indicators of emotional well-being (both directly and indirectly), it may be helpful to break out some of the major functions of work in peoples lives for further consideration. Thinking about specific functions of work rather than work as a total experience may facilitate the design of roles for older persons which will have the desired effect on their lives.

Friedmann and Havighurst's (1954) analysis of the meanings and functions of work remains one of the most useful. They identified five basic functions of work: provision of income, expenditure of time and energy, identification and status, association, and meaningful life experiences. Each of these functions is seen to potentially have several meanings in a person's life (see Table 1). Literature on older workers addresses the benefits derived from employment in each of these functional areas.

TABLE 1. Relation Between the Functions and Meanings of Work

Work Function		Work Meaning
1. Income	a)	Maintaining a minimum sustenance level of existence
	b)	Achieving some higher level or group standard
2. Expenditure of time and energy	a)	Something to do
	b)	A way of filling the day or passing time
3. Identification and status	a)	Source of self-respect
	b)	Way of achieving recognition or respect from others
	c)	Definition of role
4. Association	a)	Friendship relations
	b)	Peer group relations
	c)	Subordinate-superordinate relations
5. Source of meaningful life experiences	a)	Gives purpose to life
	b)	Creativity; self-expression
	c)	New experience
	d)	Service to others

Source: Friedman, Eugene A., and Havighurst, Robert J. *The Meaning of Work and Retirement.* Chicago: University of Chicago Press, 1954. Used by permission.

Income

The first, and perhaps most obvious, function of work is the provision of income. Friedmann and Havighurst saw this aspect of work as having meaning for workers in that it at least allows for the maintenance of a minimum sustenance level of existence or, even better, facilitates the achievement of some higher level or group standard.

Especially for low-income elderly, the income derived from employment may be a tremendous asset, not only directly in allowing them to maintain a reasonable standard of living, but also indirectly in helping them to regain a sense of control over the conditions of their life. Braver and Bowers (1977) found that the older workers employed under the Job Opportunities Program used that income primarily for essentials such as food, housing, and medical care. Their use of direct assistance programs such as Supplemental Security Income and food stamps decreased while there was a slight increase in their use of facilitative services such as transportation and senior centers. Interestingly, Braver and Bowers note that few of these low-income workers had used financial assistance programs prior to their employment. This seems to underscore the notion that we are currently dealing with cohorts of elderly who have a strong work orientation. The income produced by work may be important to them not only for what it can buy but because it allows them to continue to feel that they have earned what they have.

It is also clear, however, that people value their work for reasons other than the income it provides and that income itself has different meanings for different people. The literature commonly uses the terms "intrinsic" and "extrinsic" to differentiate the noneconomic and economic meanings of work, respectively. Extrinsic meanings are often defined to include nonpecuniary secondary gains of working such as peer association and friendship. It seems clear that the extraeconomic meanings of work are important to the elderly. In Braver and Bowers' study, for example, 70 percent of the older workers interviewed expressed a desire to continue working after they passed the income limits imposed by Social Security and 88 percent would not want to stop working even if it were financially possible. Such findings make exploration of the discrete meanings of work all the more important.

A most instructive study of the intrinsic and extrinsic meanings of work was conducted by Powers and Gandy (1971). Drawing their sample from midwestern towns of 2,500 to 10,000 population, they asked 1,900 employed men aged 50 and over whether they would quit work if they were offered the alternative of an annuity equal to their wages. In general, 70 percent of the sample said they would prefer to continue working. Those who had not yet reached retirement age were more willing to quit their job if their income was assured than were those of postretirement age. Of those who would not quit working, the reasons most commonly cited were "not believing you can get something for nothing" (40.2 percent), "enjoying of the job" (22 percent), and "feeling that life would lose its meaning" (17.6 percent).

Powers and Gandy's data suggest that different views exist about the connection between work and income among working men. At the least, there seem to be those who see work as an inescapable fact of life and cannot imagine that their situation could be otherwise, those who work primarily for the income, and a sizable group who value work for extraeconomic reasons. There is also some indication that the latter group may increase as men reach retirement age.

Various researchers have noted shifts in the relative importance of intrinsic and extrinsic valuations of work as people age but the evidence has been inconsistent as to the direction of that shift. Cohn (1979), in analyzing data from a national sample of 2,164 men and women aged 18 and over, found that the intrinsic satisfactions of work decline with age as other aspects of life become more important. He suggests that over the period of labor force participation, the satisfactions derived from work are transferred from the experience of work to its consequences (e.g., income, friendships, activity). The suggestion here is that with increasing age, work has less truly intrinsic value and, therefore, the needs it meets can be more easily addressed by alternatives such as social programs. In a similar vein, Crown (1977) reviews several studies that indicate a shift in emphasis from intrinsic to extrinsic satisfactions with work as people approach retirement. She suggests, however, that such findings may reflect a reaction to the reality of retirement policies rather than an inherent change in the ways people view their work as they age.

The work of Friedmann and Havighurst (1954) is generally closer to the findings of Powers and Gandy in its conclusion that people may initially enter the work force out of necessity but over time incorporate work as such an important part of their lives that the extraeconomic meanings take on increased importance. Friedmann and Havighurst studied workers in a wide range of occupations (steelworkers, coal miners, craftspersons, salespersons, and physicians) and, as might be expected, did find some variation according to the type of work in which the person was engaged. Those in higher status occupations tended to place more value on the noneconomic meanings of work; however, all groups of workers did recognize these meanings. Those workers who stressed the extraeconomic meanings of work were the least likely to want to retire. These researchers conclude that the meanings of work associated with the provision of meaningful life experiences, structuring of time, and peer group association can be met equally well (and at times better) by leisure time activities as by work. However, they feel that the self-respect and status associated with work involve such strong cultural definitions that a retired person is hard pressed to find substitute activities that will meet these needs. It is instructive, then, to look at the evidence to determine the extent that employment and volunteer opportunities can provide noneconomic meaning in the lives of older persons.

Expenditure of Time and Energy

The second major function of work identified by Friedmann and Havighurst involved the expenditure of time and energy, or the provision of a routine. Meanings associated with this function included having "something to do" and having a way to fill the day or pass time.

In Friedmann and Havighurst's study of preretirement aged workers, persons in all occupational groups had been found to recognize the structuring function of work. Studies of older workers have found this meaning to be of major importance. Daum, Shilkoff, and Cantor (1977), looking at a sample of 200 older workers in a Title XX program in New York City, found that 81.4 percent of these would want to work even if it were not an economic necessity. Among these subjects, 56.5 percent cited the desire to remain active and engaged as a reason for continuing to work. The importance of this motivation was of equal strength in all subgroups identified in the sample. The older workers studied by Braver and Bowers also reported valuing their work role because it provided them with a structured activity.

Lawton (1978) has stressed the importance to older people of obligatory over discretionary time use. He sees this phenomenon as being conditioned by earlier socialization and life-styles. The extent to which a particular elderly person is able to maintain the desired level of obligatory activity is influenced by cultural values, experience, health, and the availability of opportunities. Lawton feels that this preference may change over progressive cohorts as people who are more comfortable with leisure reach old age. A similar prediction was put forth by Friedmann and Havighurst, who anticipated a change in values in about 1985 when those persons born into the "economy of abundance" of the 1920s begin to reach retirement. It remains to be seen whether this prediction will be born out or whether the effects of growing up during the Depression and of the socialization provided by parents from an earlier era will be stronger influences. It does seem likely, however, that successive generations who have had more experience with leisure time and, thus, with providing structure for their own time will have decreased needs for this work function as they reach their later years. This may mean that in the future older workers and volunteers can be used more successfully in roles that demand flexibility in work schedule. To the extent that older workers are comfortable with such work patterns, their usefulness may be increased as an augmentation of the less flexible schedules of younger workers.

Identification and Status

A third function listed by Friedmann and Havighurst for work was the provision of identification and status. Meanings attached to this function were work as a source of self-respect, a way of achieving recognition or respect from others, and a source of role definition. It was these meanings that were seen as being so inherently bound up with work in our culture that no other activities could successfully substitute in providing for them. In Friedmann and Havighurst's original study, workers in all occupation groups recognized and valued this function of work.

The Special Task Force on Work in America (no date) also viewed this function of work as having primary importance. They concluded that the work role was a major shaper of identity and that the workplace was a major foci of self-evaluation. Work was seen as contributing to self-esteem by providing both a sense of mastery over self and environment and a sense of having something to offer which is of value to society. These views are well summarized by a quotation from Elliot Jacques (1961) included in the report:

> Working for a living is one of the basic activities in a man's [sic] life. By forcing him to come to grips with his environment, with his livelihood at stake, it confronts him with the actuality of his personal capacity—to exercise judgement, to achieve concrete and specific results. It gives him a continuous account of his correspondence between outside reality and the inner perception of that reality, as well as an account of the accuracy of his appraisal of himself. . . . In short, a man's work does not satisfy his material needs alone. In a very deep sense, it gives him a measure of his sanity.

The self-fulfilling prophecies that are often set up for groups such as the elderly when they accept society's limiting definitions of them has been pointed out by numerous authors (e.g., Comfort, 1976; Sarason and Lorentz, 1979). Work and volunteer roles for older people have been advocated as a way of avoiding or reversing the blows to self-esteem that can result from the major role loss imposed by retirement. Braver and Bowers, for example, reported that the older workers they studied showed increased levels of self-esteem. For some, this was attributable to their having come to feel better about themselves. For others, the critical notion was that they felt they looked better in other people's eyes. In essence, these are two ways of looking at the same dynamic: if society values those who contribute through work, then one will feel more self-respect when occupying a work role. Daum and his colleagues (1977) found only 2.5 percent of their sample of elderly Title XX employees specifically mentioning status and respect as reasons they would want to work even if it were not an economic necessity. However, when a factor analysis was performed, this motivation loaded with money (mentioned by 49.5 percent of the sample), suggesting that having an income is valued for the respect associated with it as well as for its pragmatic benefits.

Since identity and self-respect often come to be intimately associated with one's work, the loss of this role in old age can be devastating. Sainer and Zander (1971) pointed out that its effects are exacerbated in elderly who have few alternative resources on which to draw and little concept of the value of leisure time. Similar issues may arise for women who have spent much of their lives as homemakers. Even though such work is undervalued by society, it still may provide a personal sense of fulfillment and contribution. When the children (and perhaps the spouse) are gone, there is seldom a readily available alternative for channeling one's energy and desire to be of service.

The issue is often discussed in terms of role continuity (e.g., Collins and Pancoast, no date). It is generally easier for people to repackage their accustomed, self-defining roles than to completely redefine the roles that give their lives meaning. The University of Michigan's (Westerman, 1974) examination of volunteerism among older women concluded that among the motivations that bring these women into volunteer roles are the need to feel esteemed and to build self-image, the desire to "actualize" the self, the desire to perpetuate the nurturing role, and the desire to gain career experience without sacrificing equally important roles as parent and spouse. Looking at elderly volunteers in Project SERVE in Syracuse, Babic (1972) found that those volunteers often chose first to utilize previously developed skills in their assignments. Later many of them moved on to new roles when they were more comfortable with their participation in the program.

In research that looked at 100 volunteers aged 55 and over, Kaplan (1976) examined the effects on satisfaction with the volunteer role of continuity between it and former roles in the workplace, in the family, and in other volunteer settings. Of these, she found only continuity with former work roles to be associated with current volunteer role satisfaction (r = .22). Such a finding underscores the notion that work roles are the most difficult to replace in terms of their contribution to self-esteem. Kaplan felt that the volunteer roles of these older people provided the basis for role transitions, which would allow for the necessary continuity in self-defining functions.

As long as cultural values place the greatest importance on contributions that are financially rewarded and/or provided in a structured work setting, it will be difficult to replace the work role with alternative activities. Under such conditions, identity and self-respect are bound to be tied to work role for many people and the enforced role loss of retirement is a potentially damaging event.

Association

The fourth work function in Friedmann and Havighurst's scheme is association, which carries the meanings of friendship relations, peer group relations, and subordinate-superordinate relations. In short, work provides people with opportunities to be with other people of like interests and to form a variety of personal ties. Few jobs are performed in complete isolation from others. In Friedmann and Havighurst's study, this function was valued equally across all occupational groupings.

The associational function of work is one that can more easily be met through substitute activities than the function of bringing identification and status. In research exploring the meanings of "happiness," for example, Bradburn and Caplovitz (1966) found that persons who were working were the best adjusted while, for those who were not working, those with a high degree of social participation were the better adjusted.

However, work and volunteer opportunities are one good way of providing for the associational needs of the elderly and older workers appear to value this aspect of their roles. In Braver and Bowers' study, 39 percent of the older workers reported feeling less lonely since they began working. Ninety-five percent of the sample said they had found new friends through the job and 25 percent showed increased participation in community activities (likely as a result of having more friends with whom to do things). In Daum, Shilkoff, and Cantor's sample, socialization opportunities were cited by 9.5 percent of the respondents as a reason to continue working when it was no longer financially necessary. Older volunteers at the Andrus Center reported feeling less lonely and having a greater sense of support as a result of the new friendships they had formed (Seguin, 1976). Sainer and Zander (1971) found that one of the main reasons given by older persons for participating in Project SERVE was the need for social contacts. As a result, this program stressed a group approach to supervision because it served as a vehicle for facilitating peer support, social contact, and the development of friendships as well as being efficient and time saving.

In short, while the opportunities to interact with others afforded by the work/volunteer setting are an insufficient reason in themselves to open such roles to the elderly, this function is highly valued by older workers. It would be interesting to explore whether friendships associated with the workplace are valued differently by older persons than are relationships in other settings. It is possible that work-related friendships provide feedback that is more critical to identity and self-esteem because they reflect on the worker's performance in this more valued role. If so, the associational function of work may not be completely substitutable by leisure time social programs.

Source of Meaningful Life Experiences

The fifth and final work function identified by Friedmann and Havighurst is that it serves as a source of meaningful life experiences. This function gives purpose to life, allows for creativity and self-expression, provides new experiences, and allows the worker to be of service to others. The original study found that work was important to all occupational groups as an interesting, purposeful activity that is intrinsically enjoyable. The professionals in the sample (physicians) had a high awareness of its value as a means of being of service to others.

For older workers as well, it is not simply the activity of work that is important but the additional sense that one's time is being used in meaningful ways. Daum and his colleagues found that among those who would continue working beyond economic need, 26 percent mentioned the desire for meaningful life experiences as a motivating force.

The volunteers at the Andrus Center reported intellectual stimulation as one of the valued benefits of their roles. For the volunteers in Project SERVE, the second major reason given for participation (besides the need for social contacts) was the need for a useful and satisfying institutionalized role (Sainer and Zander, 1971). In a study by Ewalt and Honeyfield (1981) residents of Veteran's Administration domiciliaries who wished to remain in that institution were asked what additional resources would make their lives better. More than one-third of these men (35.3 percent) expressed a desire to have the opportunity to be helpful to other people. The authors see this finding as evidence supporting "the importance of mutuality and relatedness, of 'caring for' as well as 'being cared for', regardless of a person's apparent dependency or infirmity."

It is hardly surprising that older persons should value work as a meaningful activity. In addition to meeting the basic human need to "have a reason to get up in the morning," engagement in a useful activity increases the value of the older persons in the eyes of the community and, thus, gives them additional "trading stamps" to use in their interactions with others. In the view of exchange theorists (e.g., Dowd, 1975), the aged operate at a disadvantage in attempting to meet their needs within the larger society to the extent that they have little to offer in exchange for the goods and services they seek. Such exchanges take place constantly on the basis of power and prestige as well as concrete resources. When greater numbers of elderly are engaged in sanctioned roles that contribute to the well-being of the community, they are able to operate from a position of greater strength as they attempt to meet other needs, both as individuals and as a group. In order to effect this dynamic, the work roles of the elderly must be truly meaningful and not just "make work." Lambert, Guberman, and Morris (1964) pointed out, for example, that older persons must be convinced that they have something to contribute before they can be successfully engaged in new community roles. They are more likely to respond to specific requests for assistance than to vague suggestions that they might be able to help.

Many writers have emphasized that work not only provides a multifaceted connectedness with life for persons of all ages but for older persons it provides for a more realistic sense of connectedness in the face of the changing circumstances of their lives. The Andrus Center found, for example, that their volunteers had a broader, more realistic life outlook replacing earlier attitudes that had become obsolete under the circumstances of retirement. These older volunteers also demonstrated increased intergenerational understanding and respect and more wholesome attitudes toward retirement and their own self-worth (Seguin, 1976).

Payne (1977) refined a conceptual model for analyzing the functions of volunteer roles for the elderly. In this view, the emphasis is on recycling roles and skills in a supportive social context. In this way, Payne feels, the volunteer activity can serve to increase the older person's self-image and foster personal growth at the same time that it counteracts the negative force of social labeling of the elderly. Rose (1965) suggested that persons are most apt to acquire a group consciousness regarding their place in society as aged when they adapt to aging by seeking new roles to replace their old functions rather than by denying the aging process or by disengaging. Thus, if older persons are able to revamp the skills they bring to old age to better accommodate the realities of that stage of life, they not only are likely to maintain their own morale and self-respect but also are more apt to be able to realistically assess the position of their age group in society and to deal with those realities productively.

Operational Issues

If one concludes that the use of older workers in mental health systems is beneficial to workers, clients, and programs, then it becomes necessary to consider some of the pragmatic decisions that go into setting up a program so as to utilize the benefits of such an arrangement. Experience to date has illuminated several issues that must be considered. These include the economic constraints within which the program must operate, the relative merits of utilizing paid employees or volunteers, and the requirements for supervision, training, and support of the older workers. An additional operational issue, the basis on which tasks should be assigned, will be considered in a separate section.

Economic Constraints

To begin with, a program utilizing older workers cannot be designed without some consideration of the economic policies and programs that affect both potential workers and mental health agencies. One issue encountered early in programs in which older people are used as paid workers is the need to take into account Social Security limitations on earnings. Often, salary levels and hours of work per week are set so as to allow workers to stay within those limits. Additionally, it is often necessary to discuss the issue individually with each worker and allow the worker to make the decision as to the relative advantages and disadvantages of accruing earnings that will decrease Social Security payments. Informal arrangements regarding sick leave and vacation, for example, are used at times to assist the worker in optimizing his or her income in relation to hours worked.

A related set of problems sometimes arises regarding fringe benefits for older workers. For example, agency regulations may require that employees be provided with insurance and that they contribute to a pension plan. However, insurance agents may not allow persons over a particular age to be insured on the same basis as younger workers and both insurers and employers are often reluctant to create and pay into pension plans for employees who are unlikely to work for many years. These problems, too, are often handled by manipulation of hours of work to keep older workers below the level at which fringe benefits become available. Again, the individual worker may rightfully demand a say in such decisions.

Of course, problems of earnings limits and fringe benefits only arise if there is funding available to pay older workers for their efforts. Various factors may influence whether money will be allocated to jobs for older people. The Special Task Force to the Secretary of Health, Education and Welfare concluded in *Work in America* (no date) that use of older workers in the public sector was primarily dependent on labor supply and demand factors. Additionally, employment of older persons was seen as being reduced by a humane desire to relieve the old from physical demands, the depression era heritage of Social Security as a tool to distribute employment, the increasing numbers of elderly, a downgrading of the value of past knowledge, the relative invisibility of the old in a mobile industrial society, stereotypes of old age, and lack of awareness of the effects of unemployment on older persons. An earlier report (Breckenridge, 1953) had concluded that businesses' reluctance to hire older workers was based on concerns for the physical demands of the job and the financial burdens of pensions and insurance rather than on any lack of flexibility or lack of appreciation of the benefits of such employment practices.

Sarason and Lorentz (1979) point out that the old (along with women and the handicapped) have been seen historically as valuable during crises when human resources seem limited (e.g., World War II).

They assert that the value and supply of human resources is both defined and created socially, implying that various "crises" of the present era may also contain the potential for creative reintegration of older persons into the resource network.

Opinions differ as to the potential impact on opportunities for older workers of current economic conditions and social policies. On the one hand, high rates of unemployment (especially among young members of minority groups) mitigates against the diversion of funds to create jobs for the elderly, who are popularly viewed as "taken care of" by public programs such as Social Security. At the same time, the conservative swing in public policy advocates assistance to the needy by facilitating their employment rather than through social programming. Unfortunately, it seems likely that such a policy will emphasize encouragement of job creation within the business community rather than in public agencies, such as those of the mental health network. Some expect that the precarious nature of the economy will negate the effects of any employer motivations or public incentives to the hiring of older workers. Rosenblum (1976), for example, argues that

> marginal older workers, minority and others, have been sacrificed to prevent inflation from becoming even more rampant. The ultimate economic status of those beyond middle age, precarious at best, may come to depend more and more during the years ahead on federal employment policy rather than on the local labor markets.

It seems necessary to find ways to work within these constraints and to manipulate them to the advantage of older workers. The recent Wolfenden Report in the United Kingdom argues that unused manpower resources of older persons should be tapped through extension of the voluntary sector (*Aging International,* 1978). This may be one way to work within the realities of current social policy to bring older workers into the mental health network. Emphasis on the relatively lower cost of older workers in a time of scarcity of public dollars may also be useful.

In addition to these general economic issues, recent debate has centered on the effects of an increased retirement age. Many analyses of employment policy predict that the higher mandatory retirement age will increase employers' willingness to hire older workers since more years are available for return on such an investment (e.g., Campbell, 1979; Sheppard, 1978). It is also expected, however, that this change in policy will not motivate a substantial number of persons to work past 65 (e.g., Munro, 1977).

In short, a complex set of economic and social forces affect both the ability of mental health agencies to hire older workers and the real economic benefits that can be made available to older workers by these employers. The ways in which these issues can best be addressed in program design will likely differ at various times, but they will always need to be considered in some way.

Paid Employment versus Volunteerism

In light of the economic constraints that can affect the employment of older workers, arguments as to the relative merits of using older persons as paid employees or as volunteers become especially pertinent. This volume has generally treated the two as interchangeable on the premise that the functions and structure of the two roles are sufficiently similar that benefits and problems will be essentially the same under the two conditions. Some persons with experience in the area, however, have argued for one approach over the other.

Many persons who address this issue directly argue for remuneration of the efforts of older persons. Carp (1968), for example, as part of her study of 352 elderly public housing applicants, studied the differences between those who were working at paid jobs, those who were in volunteer roles, and those who neither worked nor volunteered. She found working elderly to be significantly better off than both volunteers and the nonworking in terms of happiness, self-image, and social relations. She concludes that, for these older persons, pay for their work is equated with self-worth. It was felt that this association might stem in part from a greater middle-aged identification being maintained by those who were working. This is in line with Trelease's findings reported in this volume, that older workers may look to employment as a means of denying their own aging. It was previously mentioned that Kaplan (1976) found satisfaction with volunteer roles among the elderly to be associated with the extent to which those roles were seen as continuous with previous work roles. In the same study, it was found that 74 percent of the older volunteers rated paid employment as having higher prestige than their volunteer role.

On the other hand, Lambert and colleagues (1964) argued that it is not monetary remuneration but the task itself that determines the prestige and status older persons derive from their work. These authors feel that prestige and gratification are inherent in the time and energy demand of the job. Others, such as Blumensohn, who has described a successful volunteer program in this volume, agree that volunteerism may in fact be more congruent with cultural values placed on altruism and contribution to the community than is paid employment.

It would be useful to study this question more closely to determine the extent to which volunteer roles fulfill the same functions for older persons as paid jobs. Economic constraints may at times make it much more possible to utilize older volunteers in the mental health system. When this is the case, it would be helpful to know whether there are certain needs that are not being as adequately addressed as they would be if the workers were paid. It would then be more possible to consider specific points of program design that could be altered to increase the meaningfulness of the volunteer roles for the older person. It would also be useful to know whether any differences in the meaning of paid and volunteer roles among the elderly impact on the ways in which they perform in these roles.

Supervision, Training, and Support

Whether a program utilizes paid or volunteer older workers, it must attend to the needs of those workers for supervision, training, and support. In essence, the agency must address cost/benefit questions regarding its staff deployment. It is necessary to provide older workers (as any other workers) with sufficient supportive input to optimize their effectiveness while at the same time avoiding burdening supervisory staff to the point that the demands on their time and energy are greater than the contributions of their new supervisees.

Clearly, some sort of supervision and/or training is required because in most cases older workers are not professionals and cannot be assigned to totally self-directed roles. Even in the case where retired professionals are utilized, at least minimal orientation to the agency and integration with its other functions is required. Additonally, however, it is important that older workers be provided with a sense of connectedness with the agency if their work is to be personally satisfying. If workers are disatisfied with their roles, the program will lose its intended effect on the well-being of the worker and may also lose the services of those workers rather quickly.

The University of Michigan's discussion of older workers (Westerman, 1974) reminds us that a successful program must include plans not only for recruitment, selection, and assignment, but also for orientation, feedback, and recognition. Kaplan (1976) found that the older volunteer's perception of the importance of his or her role was related to the extent of contact with administration, staff, and other volunteers and to the extent of integration into the agency structure. In her sample of 100 older volunteers, role satisfaction was associated with knowing the names of all or most of the agency staff, being able to consult with staff, being involved in team efforts, having shared involvements with staff, and feeling that the agency valued the volunteers' contribution. Eighty-eight percent of the volunteers felt it was important for staff and volunteers to work together. Kaplan concludes that interaction with paid staff provides external validation of the volunteer's efforts which, in turn, affirms the worth of his or her work.

Some differences of opinion exist as to the form that such interaction should take. It is generally agreed that older workers and volunteers should be approached as adult learners. In their pioneer study of the potential usefulness of paraprofessionals in social work, Barker and Briggs (1968) delineated the learning patterns of such workers in mastering case aide functions. The adult paraprofessionals they studied were found to identify with the agency, seek advice regarding specific cases and problems, learn through trial and error, seek broadening rather than deepening experiences, express more interest in questions of service delivery and standards than in theory, respond well to teaching that drew on their previous experience, learn cumulatively and deductively through their work experience, gain confidence from growing experience and from group support and teaching, and be slow to disagree with their teachers. This description of the adult learner is quite similar to that posited by Knowles (1970) to describe adult learning in general.

There is little reason to expect adult workers over age 65 to differ from this pattern in major ways and, in fact, older workers have been described in quite similar terms. Babic (1972), for example, feels that older volunteers benefit most from practical, ongoing, informal training and are somewhat intimidated by more formal training efforts. MacLean and Marcus (1979) also emphasized that older workers have been out of school for a very long time and are usually more comfortable in an informal learning setting. McCaslin and Wilson in this volume describe inductive learning patterns in their older workers that follow those attributed to the adult learner.

In general, then, it is felt that older workers benefit most from supervision and training that is informally structured, practical rather than theoretical, and based heavily on their own experience. Some writers have concluded that job-specific training upon entrance to the agency is sufficient to meet these needs (e.g., Braver and Bowers,

1977). Others, such as McCaslin and Wilson in this volume, feel that older workers value and benefit from opportunities for more general learning as long as these are provided within the framework of their adult learner patterns.

A group approach to supervision and training is sometimes advocated as an ideal way to meet both the learning needs of the older worker and the resource conservation needs of the agency. Babic (1972) feels that a group approach both provides necessary peer support and reduces the administrative time involved in utilizing older workers. Sainer and Zander (1971) attempted to test the effectiveness of group methods in recruiting, placing, training, and retaining older volunteers in community agencies. Following such methods, Project SERVE was able to place 640 volunteers in its first three years and 70 percent of these remained actively involved. Sainer and Zander interviewed 460 of these volunteers to determine the elements of the program that had been important to its success. On the basis of their data they developed the following guidelines for volunteer programs utilizing older persons:

1. The placement agencies should be assisted to develop roles appropriate to the experience and background of the older volunteers.
2. Volunteers should be placed in each agency in a group.
3. Volunteers should be offered choices regarding their placements.
4. Little training should be provided prior to placement in order to lessen the volunteers' feeling that they need to "qualify" for the positions.
5. Personal attention should be provided to the volunteers.
6. Public recongition should be provided by the community.
7. Transportation and lunch should be provided.
8. No one wanting to volunteer should be turned away.

In general, these researchers concluded that the emphasis in designing programs should be on the needs, interests, and individual differences of the volunteers rather than on the preferences of the agencies.

One other aspect of training and supervision that has been emphasized is the physical environment in which these activities take place. MacLean and Marcus (1979) argue that the learning environment is actually more important than the content of training. Seguin

(1976) pointed out that the physical environment (of work as well as training) gives the worker and others clues as to the status of the older person's role. This is in keeping with the findings of Kaplan mentioned earlier, which emphasize the worker's sensitivity to the feedback of those with whom he or she works. Additionally, the informality mentioned as an important aspect of the learning patterns of adults is facilitated by a setting that is deliberately nonreminiscent of childhood classroom experiences.

In providing for the training and supervision needs of the older worker, it cannot be forgotten that their presence places new demands on the agency and its paid staff. In fact, as McCaslin and Wilson have pointed out in this volume, older workers may have needs for personal attention and support that constitute an extra and unaccustomed demand on supervisory staff. Seguin (1976) suggested that the agency as an environment is capable of adapting to the new workers but may often resist due to the dissonance between the needs of the staff and older workers. Braver and Bowers encourage the provision of training to all workers, staff and older workers alike, to prepare them for the impact of the latter.

The impact of older workers on agency and staff is generally felt to be an issue that has to be assessed for each unique situation, taking into account the history, organization, and other demands of the agency in question. Braver and Bowers found that the agencies that were most flexible and capable of integrating older workers were those that had been in operation for 10 years or less, had a staff of 10 or less, and were either federally funded or nonprofit. The first two variables especially may underscore the need on the part of older workers for individual attention and support. Lambert and colleagues (1964) suggest that the use of a greater number of volunteers with less time contributed to the agency by each will increase requirements of supervisory and coordination time above that for the case in which fewer volunteers work for longer hours in the agency.

It appears that a number of supervisory and training patterns may be successful as long as they take into account the general needs of older workers for concrete, pragmatic guidance provided in informal settings and allowing for interaction with regular agency staff. It is equally important to the success of the program that it be designed to meet the needs of—or at least minimize the demands on—the agency and its regular staff. It will probably be useful in most cases to involve as many of the regular staff as possible in planning for the arrival of a new set of older workers. In this way their preferences can be taken into account and their investment in making the experience meaningful for the older worker increased.

Appropriate Roles for Older Workers

The programs described in this volume represented a wide range of roles and tasks through which older workers have contributed to mental health systems, including those of case aide, counselor, companion, advocate, teacher, clerical assistant, outreach worker, and opinion leader. Other writers have also advocated a range of activities for older workers. Sieder (1977), for example, suggests that older volunteers would be especially useful in outreach services to elderly clients and others, work with children, advocacy roles, and social change efforts. The University of Michigan discussion (Westerman, 1974) concluded that appropriate volunteer roles for older women included supplemental services under regular staff, enrichment programs added on to basic services, and advocacy and community bridging efforts. Program designers must make decisions as to the roles in which the potential contributions of older people would be most useful both to the agency and its clients and to the older workers themselves.

Several writers have suggested that guidelines for role design might logically flow from consideration of the realities of old age and the constraints and freedoms that life stage may bring. In this regard, Sieder (1977) reminds us that older people generally prefer to work part time and during daytime hours and that they often have transportation difficulties. Additionally, she suggests that older persons have greater needs than younger adults for opportunities for paid employment, chances to socialize with other people, and opportunities to learn, innovate, and act. Kretzmer (1976) proposes that roles that include small-group interaction and/or those that are organized so that the work is home-based may be most appropriate for meeting the socialization needs of the elderly.

If special requirements of old age are utilized as a basis for designing roles for older workers, care must also be taken that such guidelines are realistic. Especially, it is important not to overestimate the constraints imposed by old age. One National Institute of Mental Health study reported by Johnson (1976) found that, contrary to popular opinion, there was little decline in intellectual function in the middle years. Increased age was found to result in a slight reduction in reaction time and in short-term memory, but vocabulary and social intelligence were found to increase with age. A person's willingness to take risks and to make decisions in ambiguous situations decreased with advancing age. It is important that *empirical data* such as these be taken into account rather than the traditional mythology about old age, which is often a part of the views of professionals as well as lay persons.

A number of persons with experience in the use of older workers have indicated that these workers show a marked preference for tasks that involve direct client contact. The analysis of Lambert et al. (1964) notes that most older persons prefer tasks involving interpresonal communication rather than mechanical or physical tasks (including personal care). Braver and Bowers (1977) found that Title X workers in direct-service jobs had higher levels of satisfaction with their work. In Kaplan's (1976) study of elderly volunteers, common direct-service roles were seen as providing continuity with former marital and family roles. These jobs included such functions as maintaining relationships and providing reassurance and support. Continuity between these volunteer roles and former family roles was associated with satisfaction with volunteering.

Other guidelines that have been suggested for designing assignments include Wolfensberger's (1972) assertion that one should avoid the juxtaposition of socially "deviant" groups, such as in the case of old people working with the mentally retarded, as this works against attempts to normalize relations for both groups. Bristowe has raised a similar issue in this volume regarding the effects of working with the frail "old old" on the morale of the "young old." On the other hand, the program described by Schapiro offered an example of this sort of mixing of disadvantaged groups having been quite successful.

Seguin (1976) reminds us that tasks not already being carried out by other staff are both fulfilling for the older worker and nonthreatening to the regular staff. Such tasks may serve to complement staff work, fill in gaps in the organization's relations with the community, or develop new programs. She also asserts that concrete, tangible tasks more readily provide workers and others with evidence of their achievements than do ambiguous tasks. Ambiguous tasks, on the other hand, represent more of a problem-solving challenge, which may be desired by some workers.

Given the number and variety of considerations that are thought important in designing older workers' roles, it is not surprising that many writers suggest an individualized approach to worker assignment. Certainly, each agency must decide on the tasks and roles in which older persons could contribute most to its goals and functions. Beyond this, however, it is felt that individual older workers should be matched to work opportuntities on the basis of their skills, needs, education, cultural predispositions, and the meaning that work has for them (Braver and Bowers, 1977; Breckinridge, 1953; Friedmann and Havighurst, 1954; Kretzmer, 1976; Sheppard, 1976). In cases where the pool of potential workers and/or volunteers has identifiable characteristics that are relevant to their assignments, it may be possible for the agency to take these into account in designing roles so as to minimize the need for detailed assessments in actual job assignment.

Some studies have been able to differentiate the predilections and potentials of older workers on the basis of identifiable characteristics. These have included socioeconomic status, personality variables, and minority versus majority group status. Such information is helpful both for designing programs that will utilize available older workers and for guiding the process of matching workers with available jobs.

Socioeconomic Status Differences

Traditionally, volunteers of all ages have been thought of as coming from higher social classes. The assumption is that persons who seek life-enriching service opportunities will be those whose basic needs are taken care of. Likewise, it is usually expected that persons in higher status positions will be more likely to continue working into old age when this is possible. Such persons are assumed to have more investment in the personal, intrinsic satisfactions of work and to have a desire to maintain this pattern in their lives. It is recognized, of course, that lower class persons often need to continue employment into old age but their motivation is seen as largely financial and it is assumed that the nature of the job will not be an issue.

Some studies of older workers have found evidence to support these views. Daum, Shilkoff, and Cantor (1977), for example, found that among elderly Title X employees in New York City, those who saw their search for continued employment as primarily tied to the need for meaningful life experiences tended to be higher class, living with a spouse, in good health, and having been employed in a prestigious occupation. Conversely, those for whom the financial aspects of work were of primary importance had low incomes that they perceived as inadequate for meeting their needs. Ekerdt and Bosse (1977) in analyzing data from the Duke Longitudinal Study report similar findings. They note that men who do not want to retire tend to be older, married, not forced to retire, healthier, and having higher incomes, education, and occupational prestige than those who are comfortable with the notion of retirement.

At the same time, as a number of recent programs have opened up work and volunteer opportunities for older persons from lower classes, data have begun to accumulate as to the desire of a broad range of elderly to be involved in such activities. Dye and his colleagues (1973) reviewed a number of studies on older volunteers that covered a range of socioeconomic classes. In their own study of Jewish community center volunteers they found that these older people differed from nonvolunteers only in their activism patterns. Braver and Bowers (1977) note that the older workers in their sample who were most satisfied with their work role were unmarried women who had low incomes. And Bowles (1976) reports that elderly volunteers in the highly successful RSVP program had demographic characteristics much like those of older people who are usually viewed as service recipients.

Project SERVE (Sainer and Zander, 1971) was a pioneer effort at proving that lower class elderly were able and willing to fill volunteer roles. Major goals of its creators were to change the image of old age among both elderly and younger persons and to change the traditional conception of what persons are valuable as volunteers. The results of that experiment clearly showed that such efforts were needed and were an important influence in the development of federally sponsored volunteer programs, such as RSVP.

Earlier, Rosenblatt (1966) had questioned lower income, poorly educated, foreign born elderly in New York City as to their interest in volunteer opportunities. He found two groups among these to be especially interested in volunteering. These were poorly educated elderly men who were looking for new activities and better educated women who had some previous volunteer experience.

It appears, then, that elderly from all socioeconomic groups can realistically be considered as potential volunteers and workers. These groups may have somewhat different skills developed during their earlier adult years and those with lower incomes can be expected to have more need for paid employment or more need for financial assistance with the costs involved in volunteering. For example, Lambert et al. (1964), in interviewing 297 persons aged 65 and over about their ability and willingness to become involved in the activities of health agencies, found that 25 percent of the respondents would be willing and able to volunteer for free, and a little over half of these would be able to provide their own transportation. Another 15 percent of the sample would be willing to contribute if some pay were involved and somewhat more than a third would contribute to agency efforts if some assistance were provided with the costs involved. Those who were willing to be involved were not distinguishable from those who were not in terms of age, sex, health, education, previous volunteer experience, or employment status.

Personality Differences

Other researchers have attempted to identify personality character-istics that are predictive of successful involvement in work and volunteer roles for older people. Monk and Cryns (1974) analyzed desire to volunteer among white ethnic working class elderly in Buffalo. Predictors identified in this study included age, education, belief in one's ability to contribute, interest in senior citizen activities, having a range of social interests, and home ownership. In a more strictly psychological realm, those who were willing to volunteer scored high on self-perception, need for continued association with one's peers, outward-looking orientation, having self-transcendent interests, and rootedness. These researchers conclude that the achievement of integrity and generativity in old age (as described by Erikson, 1950) are associated with an orientation to be of service through volunteering.

Another study by Thune, Tine, and Booth (1964) attempted to validate selection criteria for training programs for older workers. Based on ratings from 12 trainees in Nashville (aged 63–77), employ-ability was found to be associated with tests for perserverance, Rorschach Barrier Responses, and WAIS similarities. These researchers described successful trainees as being leaders who were highly verbal and had strong ego defenses and strong personalities. The most important characteristics of the successful trainees were felt to be strong ego defenses that were mature and appropriate and a strong motivation to succeed.

Minority/Majority Group Differences

Still other investigators have tried to determine whether minority elderly must be considered differently from majority elderly in relation to work and volunteering. Jackson (1978), after examining the Harris

Poll data, concludes that race is irrelevant to retirement conditions and attitudes after socioeconomic status is controlled. It is those with low incomes, rather than minorities per se, who are more likely to want to work beyond age 65. It has been noted, however, that Mexican-American elderly more often retire as a result of poor health than other ethnic groups (Mendoza, 1978).

Minority elderly have been active in federally sponsored volunteer programs. Keller reports that minority participation is 35 percent in the Foster Grandparents Program, 44 percent in the Senior Companion Program, and 14 percent in the Retired Senior Volunteer Program (RSVP). The two former programs have more financial assistance built in than the latter, underscoring the interaction of race and low-income status. In absolute numbers, however, only about 7,000 minority elderly participate in the stipended programs and about 33,000 in RSVP. Keller suggests that minority elderly need more accessible opportunities to volunteer.

Stanford (1978), however, reminds us of a quite different issue that must be kept in mind when considering the work patterns of minority elderly. Retirement, he argues, is a relatively new concept in minority communities since in the past few elderly in these groups even reached the age of 65. Those who did live to retirement age seldom had meaningful employment from which to retire and many of them had to continue working regardless of age for economic reasons. The suggestion here is that minority elderly from lower socioeconomic groups may need more realistic opportunities to retire rather than to work or volunteer. Figures reviewed by Golden (1976) support the notion that minority elderly have been in the work force out of necessity rather than desire. He reports that from 1964 to 1974 the labor force participation of black men over age 65 declined 27 percent while that for white men decreased by only 19 percent. For older women, labor force participation from 1940 to 1974 decreased 20 percent for blacks while it increased 43 percent for whites.

Use of Older Workers as a Normalization Strategy

The literature reviewed in this chapter leaves little doubt that older workers can make significant contributions to the mental health system and, at the same time, can benefit greatly from the opportunity to make such contributions. For these reasons alone, the utilization of older workers by mental health systems appears to be a parsimonious solution to the problem of adequately addressing the community's mental health needs in a time of shrinking funds. Additionally, meeting mental health needs and problems of the elderly by facilitating their inclusion in the mainstream of community life is an approach that many theorists would consider ultimately more effective than focusing primarily on cases where breakdown has already occurred.

Most generally, the expansion of work and volunteer roles for older people is a primary prevention strategy. Caplan (1964, p. 26) defines primary prevention as a "community concept" that "involves lowering the rate of new cases of mental disorder in a population over a certain period by counteracting harmful circumstances before they have a change to produce illness." Included are attempts to modify both harmful environmental conditions and the vulnerability of persons exposed to those conditions. A central concern is the assurance that people have physical, psychosocial, and sociocultural resources that are commensurate with their stage of growth and development. The person with adequate resources will be able to maintain integrity in the face of various stress-producing crises that are inevitable in the course of life.

We have seen that work serves a variety of functions in human life. In the physical realm it provides income that is critical to the attainment of other physical resources. In the psychosocial sphere, work structures a person's expenditures of time and energy, provides opportunities for association with others, and is the source of meaningful life experiences. A major sociocultural function of work is the provision of identification and status in the community. Thus, work and volunteer opportunities have the capacity to strengthen the resources of older people in all three realms that are critical to continued mental health in the face of the many stresses that can occur in late life.[2]

More specifically, work and volunteer opportunities for older people can be viewed as a normalization strategy (Wolfensberger, 1972). The principle of normalization in mental health services had its origin in Denmark in 1959 in relation to programs for the mentally retarded and soon spread to other countries and problem areas. The normalization principle has been defined as "utilization of means which are as culturally normative as possible, in order to establish and/ or maintain personal behaviors and characteristics which are as culturally normative as possible" (Wolfensberger, p. 28). Basically, the notion is that if a group of people are labeled as a client group and singled out for special attention, it is easy to begin thinking of them as fundamentally different from other people. Rather than feed into this self-fulfilling prophesy in which those in the client group begin to think of themselves as dependent and to act accordingly, programs designed according to a normalization principle attempt to create a "positive self-fulfilling prophesy." Services and treatment are geared to making the lives of the client group as much like that of everyone else as possible.

The increased inclusion of older people in contributory roles in the mainstream of community activities clearly functions to meet several of their basic needs without identifying the elderly as a dependent client group. Thus, not only are important needs met, but problems of self-labeling and dependency on service are avoided. Stereotypes of older people held by the general populace may be affected, thus reducing other stresses experienced by the aged that stem from an ubiquitous social devaluation.

Such approaches are also in keeping with principles of helping followed by professional social workers within the mental health system. Meyer (1976), for example, is a major spokesperson for an individualized approach to social work practice that pays attention to the environment within which the client and his or her problem exist. A major strategy in her theory is the identification of "life-space" opportunities for intervention. In other words, the professional design-ing services should look for situations in which persons may be found who are under stress but have not yet broken down or even identified their stresses as unusual enough to warrant personal attention. An employment agency or volunteer placement bureau for older persons is an excellent example of the life-space situation Meyer describes. Here one finds large numbers of elderly people who are looking for a solution to one or more of the stresses associated with retirement. Most of these persons will benefit from the job or voluntary opportunity they are seeking. Additionally, some of them will need other sorts of assistance including psychotherapeutic intervention. The employment agency, therefore, can serve as both a major preventive service and a case-finding opportunity that has the capacity to channel older persons into the mental health system sooner than would otherwise be the case.[3]

Meyer lists four guiding principles for social work practice that seem to fit well the notion of increasing work opportunities for the elderly as a mental health strategy:

1. *To serve as many people as quickly and parsimoniously as possible.* Less professional time is involved in matching individuals with jobs than in providing traditional mental health services. Assuming sufficient jobs are available, then, more older persons can be helped more quickly. Additionally, we have seen that multiple needs can be met through this one service.

2. *To view individuals in their natural life situation as part of a transactional field of person-in-environment.* The provision of work opportunities for the aged recognizes the dependence of the individual on the environment for resources to meet a variety of needs. The solution is also framed in terms of effecting a more mutually supportive relation between the individual and the community.

3. *To provide for reestablishment of psychosocial balance rather than for "long-term" therapeutic efforts at "cure."* Work and volunteer opportunities correct the imbalance in the immediate situation rather than searching for inadequacies within the individual that have played into his or her adverse reaction to retirement. The latter approach may be necessary and appropriate in some cases but the more immediate solution should be attempted first because it will be helpful to the largest number of persons.

4. *To intervene directly to strengthen individual coping mechanisms and to reinforce social supports.* Employment of meaningful volunteer roles can augment the supports necessary to older persons in several areas. To the extent that these supportive resources are increased, the coping capacity of the individual will be enhanced. Given the numerous stresses that can occur in old age, multiple supportive resources are essential for continued, flexible adaptation.

Yet another theoretical view that is helpful in understanding the potential importance of employment strategies with older people is the notion of "empowerment" explored by Solomon (1976). In this view, the issue of powerlessness is seen as central in working with members of oppressed groups. Although Solomon's thesis was developed in relation to social work practice in the black community, it seems easily adaptable to consideration of the problems of the elderly.[4]

Solomon differentiates power blocks in terms of their source and impact as being either direct or indirect. Direct power blocks are those "based on negative valuation that have not been incorporated into the developmental experiences of the individual but are applied directly by some agent of society's major social institutions" (p. 18). By definition, these power blocks are most pertinent to the situation of the aged since old age has not been experienced throughout the development of the individual. Rather, the elderly person is facing for the first time a socially imposed devaluation based on the number of years he or she has lived.

Direct power blocks can occur at three levels. Primary direct power blocks involve inadequate services or resources for the group as a whole. The scarcity of job opportunities for the elderly falls into this category. Secondary direct power blocks come from a lack of opportunities for the individual to develop skills needed for coping. When an older person is forced to retire, for example, his or her development as a skilled employee is stopped although the need to be capable of contributing to the community continues to the end of life. Tertiary direct power blocks, finally, occur when valued social roles are denied to people (or the resources necessary to performance in some role). At this level, the status and identification functions of work come to mind. For many people, to be barred from work is to be denied a sense of social worth.

Indirect power blocks, being based on developmental influences, are less relevant to the situation of the elderly, except perhaps at the tertiary level. Here Solomon speaks of the effect of limited personal resources and skills in decreasing the individual's effectiveness in performing socially valued roles. In addition to the deficits that may accompany increasing age, removal from the labor force will, in time, cause the older person's previously developed skills to decline or to become outdated. Thus, the elderly individual's capacity to reenter the job maket will often decrease over time.

Solomon suggests three major roles that practitioners may undertake in order to effectively intervene with groups of people who are in a position of powerlessness. First, the practitioner may act as a resource consultant, augmenting the client's knowledge of sources of assistance and his or her capacity to utilize those that do exist. Making older persons aware of work and volunteer opportunities that do exist (and helping to create such opportunities) is a good example of this approach. Second, the practitioner may act as a sensitizer, helping clients to gain the self-knowledge necessary to solve their problems. For example, a mental health professional might help a retired man to understand the ways in which his ceasing to work has created his current depression and encourage him to take on a voluntary assignment as a means of reestablishing his self-esteem. Finally, the practitioner may take on the role of teacher/trainer, guiding the process through which the clients enhance their coping capacity. Employment agencies and volunteer placement services for the elderly often take on such responsibilities. Older persons may need some retraining in order to take advantage of opportunities and/or they may need assistance in preparing for the process of applying for a job for the first time in many years (and for the first time as an "older worker"). In all three approaches, the focus is on "empowering" the client, i.e., the primary purpose is to enable the individual to solve his or her own problems. Certainly, moving older persons back into contributory roles helps to put them back in control of their own lives. In many cases, their capacity to work out other problematic situations in their lives will be enhanced as a result of increased self-confidence and self-esteem.

In addition to these practitioner roles, Solomon advocates the use of the client as a service provider as a powerful empowerment strategy. This strategy is seen as potentially bringing about a more equal relationship between professional and client, which mitigates against reinforcement of the client's position of helplessness. Simply put, those who contribute to others not only respect themselves more but expect (and usually receive) more respect from others. This notion is central to the idea of utilizing the talents of older workers within the mental health system.

Whether we look at the use of older workers in the mental health system in terms of normalization or empowerment or any of a number of other theoretical perspectives, its power as an effective stragegy for enhancing the mental health of the elderly is evident. It is possible, in fact, that only approaches that provide for real contributions by the elderly will be effective in overcoming the negative psychological effects of forced retirement. Rosow (1967) in exploring the mutual assistance patterns of the elderly concludes that there may be no effective substitute for a major role loss in old age except an equally significant status that is valued and rewarded. Work is so central to adult identity that alternate uses of time, such as leisure activities, may be ineffective in replacing it.

Recognition and use of the unique skills and talents of the elderly by the mental health system assists older people to utilize their strengths to solve their own problems rather than focusing on their weaknesses and treating them as a group that will necessarily be dependent. It is a mental health strategy that has the power to reverse stereotypes of old age that are a source of multiple stresses, adversely affecting the mental health of individual older persons.

Need for Further Research

A considerable amount of information has accrued in a relatively short time regarding the use of older workers in mental health systems and in related jobs. Certainly, enough experience has come from programs such as those described in this volume that agencies can initiate projects using older persons with a fair degree of certainty as to the results. However, certain critical questions remain unanswered that may be important in optimizing the effectiveness and efficiency of future efforts in this area. Hopefully, new programs will be sensitive to these issues and will build in research strategies to add to our understanding, while at the same time researchers will seek out opportunities to study both new and existing older worker projects in the mental health system.

Seguin (1976) provides a useful framework for considering these unanswered questions, categorizing them as having to do with either the worker, the work-setting or the work. That typology is used below with appropriate modifications to include the concerns of programs utilizing paid workers as well as those drawing on older persons as volunteers.

The Worker

In this category, Seguin poses the question, "Under what conditions will retired individuals take on positions in work-oriented organizations, or reject them? Continue or discontinue in them?" Older persons may seek the familiar from their adult lives in the workplace and the roles associated with it, or they may choose to avoid such settings and tasks and turn instead to new experiences in their later years. The evidence suggests that older persons who do work place a high value on continuity in their lives. The question remains, however, whether such elderly differ from their peers on this dimension or whether the search for continuity is universal and older persons differ instead in terms of their opportunities to realize this goal. More studies must be conducted with cross-sections of the older population—workers and nonworkers alike—to examine in greater depth the life situations, personality characteristics, and desires of these two groups.

A related question that has been raised in this book is whether there is a difference between older persons who volunteer and those who seek paid employment. Existing data suggest that earned income is closely tied to status and prestige in Western culture and that these functions of work are of major importance to older people. However, we also know that large numbers of older persons engage in voluntary pursuits and derive substantial benefits from these activities. Again, one must ask whether older paid workers and volunteers differ in some significant way or whether the two groups are simply taking advantage of the opportunities available to them. It would be important to know if different types of older people are more suitable for the different roles. Programs could then be designed taking into account the available pool of workers and/or volunteers, and recruitment efforts could be better targeted.

The Work-Setting

In this category, Seguin asks, "Under what conditions will organizations use older workers and/or volunteers or reject such personnel?" We have reviewed literature indicating that certain types of agencies are more responsive to hiring older workers than others and better able to adjust to their presence. It would be helpful not only to better understand these agency differences but also to be able to identify the specific issues that make hiring older persons problematic for some. It might then be possible to redesign programs so that they will work in settings where standard models are resisted.

Seguin also draws our attention to the response of the worker to the work setting. She cites Pitterman's (1973) enumeration of factors that can satisfy the older volunteer's need to avoid pain from the environment: organizational policies and administrative practices, kind of supervision under which the person works, working conditions, interpersonal relations and supports maintained for the worker, and the amount of status, security, and pay that the person accrues for doing the work. It is clear from the literature that the work setting makes a difference in the satisfaction the older person derives from his or her job. It is less clear which factors are most important and what environmental problems will result in the older worker's leaving the work-setting. There are also no comparisons in this regard of the environmental needs of paid workers as opposed to volunteers. Are paid workers, for example, more willing to put up with minor discomforts in the work setting because of the offsetting value of the income they receive? Answers to these questions would be especially helpful in reducing worker turnover and, therefore, optimizing the benefits of time and resources devoted to training new workers.

The Work

In this final area, Seguin asks, "What kinds of positions can older workers and volunteers take or create? What are the new or modified roles they enact from them?" We have seen that older workers as a group are capable of successfully filling and deriving satisfaction from a wide range of roles. We have also noted, however, that there is incomplete and at times contradictory evidence as to what types of older persons do best in specific assignments. This is perhaps the most crucial area in which additional research is needed as it has implications for efficient recruitement, design of training, and successful retention of older workers and volunteers.

We need to look further at both demographic characteristics and personality attributes that make for successful engagement in various types of work roles. Wherever possible, these variables need to be measured in such a way that they can be translated into screening questions for use in the recruitment process. It may be helpful also to look at variations in jobs of a general type that make for greater or lesser success for older as opposed to younger employees so that such differences can be taken into account in program design. In this area, too, there may be differences in the roles that are most appropriate for paid workers and volunteers.

It is quite likely that variables from these three categories interact on many issues. It would be most useful to conduct larger studies that can cover a greater range of types of workers, work settings, and work roles in order to arrive at more specific formulae for successful program design and operation. The more older persons are utilized in mental health settings, the more possible this sort of inquiry will become.

Conclusion

The idea of older persons working is not new. Such an issue could only arise in contemporary society in which persons over a certain age are defined out of the work force. Perhaps we are only now to the point of having sufficient experience with universal retirement to have become aware of the problems that not working can pose for the elderly.

It appears that the time has come to seriously consider ways of reintegrating older persons into the mainstream as contributing members of society. To deny them such roles is potentially to do serious damage to their mental health. What better place, then, to begin the needed reversal of policy than in the mental health system itself?

Older workers have unique and valuable contributions to make to the mental health system, including providing effective and dependable service, humanizing services, facilitating expansion of and innovation in programs, contributing well-developed skills and extensive life experience, enhancing the agency's public relations, reaching clients who are distrustful of younger professionals, and contributing to a reduced service need for themselves and other elderly. At the same time, their involvement in work roles enhances their own mental health by augmenting their coping resources in the physical, psychosocial, and sociocultural realms. Work provides increased income, structure for a person's time and energy expenditure, opportunities for association with others, meaningful life experiences, and identification and status in the community.

In short, the utilization of older workers in the mental health system is an effective and efficient primary prevention strategy. It enhances older persons' well-being so that they can avoid breakdown rather than waiting for the stresses to take their toll and then engaging costly resources in rehabilitation. The impact of such a strategy can go far beyond the individual elderly who are employed. The presence of functional older people in the agency contributing meaningfully to the needs of the community can convey a powerful message to all people and help to reverse the negative stereotypes that lead to innumerable unnecessary stresses in the lives of all older people. Perhaps most important, the use of older workers in the mental health system serves to engage them in creating the solutions to their own problems—it "reempowers" the devalued elderly. Thus, the elderly become partners with professionals in advancing their interests rather than being passive recipients or objects of our study and treatment.

The obstacles to use of older workers is primarily economic. In a time of scarce resources we must push hard for the allocation of funds to those projects which we feel should have the highest priority. Surely the well-being of the most rapidly growing segment of the population deserves priority consideration? And surely a society facing resource scarcity cannot afford to continue to waste resources that can be obtained from such a large segment of its citizenry? Even in a time of austerity in government spending it is easy to argue for the use of older persons in service roles as an answer to some of our problems.

Older persons are able and willing to be part of the answer, not only to their own problems but also to the problems of other members of the community. They lack only the opportunity. Opportunities created for older workers to serve in the mental health system are opportunities for many people to have a better life—both now and in their own old age.

Notes

1. Sussman (1977) applied this model to analysis of the interactions between older persons and their families.
2. Differences that have been noted among older persons in the degree to which they value the various functions of work may be, in part, a function of the differences among the needs of these individual elderly. For example, a low-income person would be expected to place a high value on the economic functions of work. Similarly, an elderly person who is isolated from family and friends might give top priority to the associational functions of employment.
3. The latter would be seen as an early interventive approach (Caplan, 1964).
4. The similarities and differences between the situation of ethnic minorities and that of the aged has been explored by such scholars as Rose (1968) and Streib (1968).

References

Babic, A. L. The older volunteer: Expectations and satisfactions. *The Gerontologist*, 1971, *12*, 87–90.
Barker, R. L., and Briggs, T. L. *Differential Use of Social Work Manpower*. New York: National Association of Social Workers, 1968.
Bowles, E. Older persons as providers of services: Three federal programs. In F. Riessman (ed.), *Older Persons: Unused Resources for Unmet Needs*. Beverly Hills: Sage, 1976.
Bradburn, N. with the assistance of E. Edward Noll. *The Structure of Psychological Well-Being*. Chicago: Aldine, 1969.
Braver, R. C., and Bowers, L. A. *The Impact of Employment Programs on the Older Worker and the Service Delivery Systems: Benefits Derived and*

Provided. Washington, D.C.: Foundation for Applied Research, June 30, 1977.

Breckinridge, E. L. *Effective Use of Older Workers.* New York: Wilcox and Follett, 1953.

Briefs: Volunteers. *Aging International,* 1978, *5,* 14.

Campbell, S. Delayed mandatory retirement and the working woman. *The Gerontologist,* 1979, *19,* 257–263.

Caplan, G. *Principles of Preventive Psychiatry.* New York: Basic Books, 1964.

Carp, F. M. Differences among older workers, volunteers, and persons who are neither. *Journal of Gerontology,* 1968, *23,* 497–501.

Carter, H. A. The retired senior citizen as a resource to minimize underachievement of children in public schools. *Archives of Physical Medicine and Rehabilitation,* 1964, *45,* 218–223.

Cohn, Richard M. Age and the satisfactions from work. *Journal of Gerontology,* 1979, *34,* 264–272.

Collins, A. H. and Pancoast, D. L. *Natural Helping Networks: A Strategy for Prevention.* Washington, D.C.: National Association of Social Workers, no date.

Comfort, A. Age prejudice in America. In F. Riessman (ed.), *Older Persons: Unused Resources for Unmet Needs.* Beverly Hills: Sage, 1976.

Crown, S. M. Morale, careers, and personal potentials. In J. E. Birren and K. W. Schaie (eds.), *Handbook of the Psychology of Aging.* New York: Van Nostrand Reinhold, 1977.

Daum, M., Shilkoff, M. L., and Cantor, M. H. The meaning of work for re-employed older workers. Paper presented at the 30th Annual Scientific Meeting of the Gerontological Society, San Francisco, November 1977.

Dowd, J. J. Aging as exchange: A preface to theory. *Journal of Gerontology,* 1975, *30,* 584–594.

Dye, D., Goodman, M., Roth, M., Bley, N., and Jensen, K. The older adult volunteer compared to the nonvolunteer. *The Gerontologist,* 1973, *13,* 215–218.

Ekerdt, D. J., and Bosse, R. Rejection of retirement. Paper presented at the 30th Annual Scientific Meeting of the Gerontological Society, San Francisco, November 1977.

Erikson, E. H. *Childhood and Society,* 2nd Ed. New York: W. W. Norton, 1950.

Ewalt, P. L., and Honeyfield, R. M. Needs of persons in longterm care. *Social Work,* 1981, *26,* 223–231.

Friedmann, E. A., and Havighurst, R. J. *The Meaning of Work and Retirement.* Chicago: University of Chicago Press, 1954.

Golden, H. M. Black ageism. In F. Riessman (ed.), *Older Persons: Unused Resources for Unmet Needs.* Beverly Hills: Sage, 1976.

Gray, R. M., and Kasteler, J. M. An evaluation of the effectiveness of a foster grandparent project. *Sociology and Social Research,* 1970, *54,* 181–189.

Jackson, J. J. Retirement patterns of aged blacks. In E. P. Stanford (ed.),

Retirement: Concepts and Realities. San Diego: University Center on Aging, San Diego State University, 1978.

Jacques, E. *Equitable Payment*, 1961. Cited in Special Task Force to the Secretary of Health, Education, and Welfare, *Work in America*. Cambridge, Mass.: MIT Press, no date.

Johnson, J. M. Is 65+ Old? In F. Reissman (ed.), *Older Persons: Unused Resources for Unmet Needs*. Beverly Hills: Sage, 1976.

Kaplan, B. I. Role continuity and satisfaction in the volunteer role. Paper presented at the 29th Annual Scientific Meeting of the Gerontological Society, New York, October 1976.

Keller, J. B. Volunteer activities for ethnic minority elderly. In E. P. Stanford (ed.), *Retirement: Concepts and Realities*. San Diego: University Center on Aging, San Diego State University, 1978.

Kent, D. P. Changing welfare to serve minority aged. In *Minority Aged in America*. Ann Arbor: Institute on Gerontology, University of Michigan, Occasional Paper #10, 1971.

Knowles, M. S. *The Modern Practice of Adult Education: Andragogy Versus Pedagogy*. New York: Association Press, 1970.

Kretzmer, M. *Guide to Israeli Research in Social Gerontology*. Jerusalem: Brookdale Institute, 1976.

Lambert, C., Jr., Guberman, M., and Morris, R. Reopening doors to community participation for old people: How realistic? *Social Service Review*, 1964, *38*, 42–50.

Lawton, M. P. Leisure activities for the aged. *Annals of the American Academy of Political and Social Science*, 1978, *438*, 71–80.

Litwak, E. Agency and family linkages in providing neighborhood services. In D. Thursz and J. L. Vigilante (eds.), *Reaching People: The Structure of Neighborhood Services*. Beverly Hills: Sage, 1978.

MacLean, M., and Marcus, L. The role of senior consultants in an aging course Paper presented at the Fifth Anniversary Meeting of the Association for Gerontology in Higher Education, Washington, D.C., March 1979.

Mendoza, L. The role and value of the Latino natural helper in retirement. In E. P. Stanford (ed.), *Retirement: Concepts and Realities*. San Diego: University Center on Aging, San Diego State University, 1978.

Meyer, C. H. *Social Work Practice: The Changing Landscape*, 2nd Ed. New York: Free Press, 1967.

Meyer, H. J. Professionalization and the nonprofessional: A sociological analysis. Paper presented at the National Association of Social Workers—American Psychological Association Conference on the Utilization of Nonprofessionals in Mental Health Work, May 1967. Quoted in R. L. Barker and T. L. Briggs, *Differential Use of Social Work Manpower*. New York: National Association of Social Workers, 1968.

Monk, A., and Cryns, A. G. Predictions of voluntaristic intent among the aged. *The Gerontologist*, 1974, *14*, 425–429.

Munro, D. R. Social Security and elderly labor supply. Paper presented at the 30th Annual Scientific Meeting of the Gerontological Society, San Francisco, November 1977.

Palmore, E. (ed.). *Normal Aging: Reports from the Duke Longitudinal Study, 1955–1969.* Durham, N.C.: Duke University Press, 1970.

Payne, B. P. The older volunteer: Social role continuity and development. *The Gerontologist,* 1977, *17*, 355–361.

Pearl, A. Youth in lower class settings. Paper presented at the Fifth Symposium on Social Psychology, Norman, Oklahoma, 1964. Cited in Bowles, Older persons as providers of services: Three federal programs. In F. Riessman (ed.), *Older Persons: Unused Resources for Unmet Needs.* Beverly Hills: Sage, 1976.

Pitterman, L. *The Older Volunteer: Motivation to Work.* Prepared for Older American Volunteer Project/ACTION, Washington, D.C., 1973.

Powers, E. A., and Gandy, W. J. Examination of the meaning of work to older workers. *International Journal of Aging and Human Development,* 1971, *2*, 38–45.

President's Commission on Mental Health. *Report to the President,* Vol. 1. Washington, D.C.: U.S.Gov. Printing Office, 1978.

Rose, A. M. Group consciousness among the aging. In A. M. Rose and W. A. Peterson (eds.), *Older People and Their Social World.* Philadelphia: F. A. Davis, 1965.

Rose, A. M. The subculture of the aging: A topic for sociological research. In B. L. Neugarten (ed.), *Middle Age and Aging,* Chicago: University of Chicago Press, 1968.

Rosenblatt, A. Interest of older people in volunteer activities. *Social Work,* 1966, *11*, 87–94.

Rosenblum, M. J. Hard times hit the old hardest. In F. Reissman (ed.), *Older Persons: Unused Resources for Unmet Needs.* Beverly Hills: Sage, 1976.

Rosow, I. *Social Integration of the Aged.* New York: Free Press, 1967.

Sainer, J., and Zander, M. Guidelines for older person volunteers. *The Gerontologist,* 1971, *11*, 201–204.

Sarason, S. B., and Lorentz, E. *The Challenge of the Resource Exchange Network.* San Francisco: Jossey-Bass, 1979.

Seguin, M. M. *Releasing the Potential of the Older Volunteer.* Los Angeles: Ethel Percy Andrus Gerontology Center, University of Southern California, 1976.

Sheppard, H. L. Work and retirement. In R. H. Binstock and E. Shanas (eds.), *Handbook of Aging and the Social Sciences.* New York: Van Nostrand Reinhold, 1976.

Sheppard, H. L. The issue of mandatory retirement. *Annals of the American Academy of Political and Social Sciences,* 1978, *438*, 40–49.

Sieder, V. M. Older persons as a resource in our society. Paper presented at the 5th National Association of Social Workers Symposium, San Diego, November 1977.

Solem, P. E. Paid work after retirement age, and mortality. Paper presented at the 30th Annual Scientific Meeting of the Gerontological Society, San Francisco, November 1977. Abstracted in *Ageing International,* 1978, 5, 20.

Solomon, B. B. *Black Empowerment: Social Work in Oppressed Communities.* New York: Columbia University Press, 1976.

Special Task Force to the Secretary of Health, Education and Welfare. *Work in America.* Cambridge, Mass.: MIT Press, no date.

Stanford, E. P. Perspectives on ethnic elderly retirement. In E. P. Stanford (ed.), *Retirement: Concepts and Realities.* San Diego: University Center on Aging, San Diego State University, 1978.

Streib, G. F. Are the aged a minority group? In B. L. Neugarten (ed.), *Middle Age and Aging.* Chicago: University of Chicago Press, 1968.

Streib, G., and Streib, R. B. Retired persons and their contributions: Exchange theory. Paper presented at the 11th International Congress of Gerontology, Tokyo, August 1978.

Sussman, M. B. Family, bureaucracy, and the elderly individual: An organizational/linkage perspective. In E. Shanas and M. B. Sussman (eds.), *Family, Bureaucracy, and the Elderly.* Durham, N.C.: Duke University Press, 1977.

Thune, J., Tine, S., and Booth, F. E. Retraining older adults for employment in community services. *The Gerontologiest,* 1964, 4, 5–9.

Thursz, D., and Vigilante, J. L. *Reaching People: The Structure of Neighborhood Services.* Beverly Hills: Sage, 1978.

Westerman, M. P. (reporter). Volunteerism. In *No Longer Young: The Older Woman in America.* Ann Arbor: Institute of Gerontology, University of Michigan, 1974.

Wolfensberger, W. *Normalization: The Principle of Normalization in Human Services.* Toronto: National Institute on Mental Retardation (through Leonard Crainford Toronto), 1972.

Wylie, M. Life satisfaction as a program impact criterion. *Journal of Gerontology,* 1970, 25, 36–40.

Index

DATE DUE

GAYLORD

PRINTED IN U.S.A.